# REPRODUCTIVE HEALTH

*The Missing Millennium Development Goal*

# REPRODUCTIVE HEALTH

## *The Missing Millennium Development Goal*

Poverty, Health, and Development in a Changing World

Arlette Campbell White
Thomas W. Merrick
Abdo S. Yazbeck

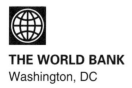

**THE WORLD BANK**
Washington, DC

ISBN-10: 0-8213-6613-0          e-ISBN: 0-8213-6614-9
ISBN-13: 978-0-8213-6613-4      DOI: 10.1596/978-0-8213-6613-4

*Library of Congress Cataloging-in-Publication Data has been applied for.*

# Contents

## FIGURES

## TABLES

## BOXES

# Foreword

Recent research findings about persistent inequality in health outcomes and the use of health services in a large number of low- and middle-income countries have raised serious policy questions about the causes and what can be done to address them. These questions are amplified when considering reproductive health. As this book finds, not only are health and support sectors, such as education and infrastructure, failing the poor and socially vulnerable, but this failure is at its worst for poor women. Too many poor women die while giving birth, suffer from malnutrition, are victims of violence, and are denied very basic rights and services.

This book, and the World Bank Institute's Learning Program it is based on, has as an ultimate objective the empowerment of key actors in the Reproductive Health community working on the ground to improve outcomes and address inequalities. The tools presented in this book are mainly applied knowledge and skills that strengthen the ability of reproductive health champions to understand the determinants of outcomes, analyze the constraints at the household and community levels, understand and address cultural factors, measure and counteract inequalities, recognize and take account of political economy factors, understand and address the impact of demographic and epidemiological transitions, improve costing and budgeting, engage in prioritization, and influence health sector reform.

The main message behind the book and the WBI program on this topic is that while disease-specific global initiatives in health, health sector reforms, and new financial aid modalities can be seen as challenges for the reproductive health agenda, hard work and building country-based skills can turn them into opportunities for improving health outcomes and building supporting systems.

I am pleased to see that this book presents diverse examples of how one can build capacity for countries to meet their reproductive health objectives through bettering the skills of health practitioners, improving access to global knowledge and ideas and customizing them into skills and tools for country-based engagement, and supporting large-scale societal change through advocacy on attitudes toward women and health, which can drive deeper change for higher impact at the country level.

I fully support the call the book makes to the global reproductive health community to continue to strengthen the empirical evidence for reproductive health and to invest in building capacity at the national and subnational levels for turning evidence-based knowledge into positive reproductive health outcomes, especially for the poor and vulnerable.

*Frannie Léautier*
*Vice President, World Bank Institute*
*The World Bank*

# Acknowledgments

The genesis of this book was a World Bank Institute course that was developed in 1998 as a response to the International Conference on Population and Development (ICPD), held in Cairo in 1994 and commonly referred to as the "Cairo conference" thereafter. The course—then titled "Adapting to Change" and retitled "Achieving the MDGs: Reproductive Health, Poverty Reduction, and Health Sector Reform" in 2002—was developed collaboratively by the World Bank, the World Health Organization (WHO), the United Nations Population Fund (UNFPA), the Joint United Nations Programme on HIV/AIDS (UNAIDS), and technical staff from other agencies. The course and the learning program that followed—including its adaptation to Africa, Latin America, and South Asia—received financial support from the World Bank Institute and from the governments of the Netherlands, the United Kingdom, Switzerland, Sweden, Norway, Finland, Ireland, Canada, and the United States of America, as well as from the Hewlett Foundation, the Packard Foundation, and the Rockefeller Foundation. The authors thank the technical and funding partners for their support.

The authors also thank many World Bank and partner agency staff and consultants who built the content base for this course and this book. At the risk of forgetting a few, here is a list of the technical and operational contributors over the past eight years, beginning with those from outside the World Bank: Carla AbouZahr, Jere Behrman, Marge Berer, David Bloom, John Bongaarts, Margaret Catley-Carlson, Tessie Catsambas, Allan Hill, Allen Kelley, Jim Knowles, Kathy Krasovec, Charlotte Leighton, Barbara McPake, Marc Mitchell, Michael Reich, Koen Rossel-Cambier, Fred Sai, Marsha Slater, and Freddie Ssengooba. From within the Bank, we thank Mark Blackden, Ed Bos, Jean Jacques de St. Antoine, Gilles Dussault,

Okubagzhi Gebreselassie, Julian Harris, Meri Helleranta, Jo Hindriks, Edna Jonas, Lan Joo, Hadia Karam, Marlilyn Lauglo, Elizabeth Lule, Tazim Mawji, John May, Don McDonald, Marguerite Monnet, Norbert Mugwagwa, David Peters, Laura Raney, Khama Rogo, Paul Shaw, Gaston Sorgho, Elizabeth Szollosi, Anne Tinker, Debrework Zewdie, and Caroline Zwicker.

Over the past eight years, the course has been offered over 15 times in Washington, Turin, Bangkok, as well as in regional and country adaptations in Africa, Latin America, and South Asia. The authors thank the large group of course alumni who provided valuable feedback and encouraged us to write the book. It is the commitment and dedication of our course participants that have made the learning program a labor of love and guided us in the development of this book.

The authors thank the editorial, production, and marketing team at the World Bank's Office of the Publisher for their high-quality work and for their invaluable guidance to improve and complete the book. Thanks to *Reproductive Health Matters* for permission to reprint elements of two journal articles authored by two of the co-authors.

Finally, the learning program that led to this book benefited from technical and operational partnerships with a variety of training institutions around the world. Our global courses gained from partnerships with Harvard School of Public Health, the International Labour Organization training program in Turin, and Chulalongkorn University in Bangkok. Our regional partners in Africa and Latin America include the African Population Advisory Council; African Medical Research and Education Foundation; Association Burkinabé de Santé Publique, Burkina Faso; Centre Africain d'Etudes Supérieures en Gestion, Sénégal; Centre d'Etudes de la Famille Africaine, Togo; Centre d'Etudes et de Recherche sur la Population pour le Développement, Mali; Centre de Formation en Santé de la Famille, Burkina Faso; Centre de Formation et de Recherche en Matiére de Population, Benin; Centre de Formation et de Recherche en Santé de la Reproduction, Sénégal; Commonwealth Regional Health Community Secretariat, Tanzania; Eastern and Southern African Management Institute, Tanzania; Fundacion Mexicana para la Salud; Intellfit African Training Centre Inc., Nigeria; Mauritius Institute of Health; Packard Foundation, Addis Ababa; The Population Council, Kenya and Mexico; and Université Cheikh Anta Diop, Sénégal.

# *Abbreviations*

| | |
|---|---|
| ANC | antenatal care |
| BIA | benefit incidence analysis |
| BOD | burden of disease |
| CPIA | Country Policy and Institutional Assessment |
| CQC | costing quality checklist |
| DHS | Demographic and Health Surveys |
| FGM/C | female genital mutilation/cutting |
| FP | family planning |
| ICPD | International Conference on Population and Development |
| IMR | infant mortality rate |
| MBB | marginal budgeting for bottlenecks |
| MCH | maternal and child health |
| MDGs | Millennium Development Goals |
| MMR | maternal mortality ratio |
| PHR | Partners for Health Reform |
| RH | reproductive health |
| SNA | System of National Accounts |
| STIs | sexually transmitted infections |
| VCCT | voluntary and confidential counseling and testing |

# PART I

## *Reproductive Health in a Changing World*

# 1

## *Twelve Years since Cairo: Blurry Vision and a Stark Reality*

A key feature of the 1994 International Conference on Population and Development (ICPD) Program of Action was a move toward a holistic approach to reproductive health. The program framers envisioned a health system and a social structure that make choices available and that address difficult cultural issues, such as female genital mutilation and other forms of violence against women. The program agenda was broad, by design, and covered a variety of services to be delivered by systems extending across sectors and social domains.

### A Broad and Ambitious Agenda under Attack

Critical to the success of the ICPD's ambitious Program of Action agenda is national and global political will to address taboos and provide the resources needed to strengthen systems to deliver an expanded set of services. Some early successes gave the reproductive health community hope. In Bangladesh, for example, the government and a large consortium of donors agreed on an ambitious program that (1) prioritized reproductive health, (2) designed patient-centered services, (3) committed large shares of public resources to essential services, (4) unified health and family planning wings of service delivery, (5) widened participation by civil society and women's groups, (6) mainstreamed gender issues, (7) addressed men and women in family planning programs and recognized side effects of contraceptives, and (8) treated violence against women as a public health issue. A change in government, however, brought about reversals in critical policy areas such as unification of the service delivery of the Ministry of Health's health and family planning wings (Jahan 2003).

Twelve years after its articulation, the ICPD agenda has lost momentum. One reason is that the act of signing on to the agenda has not automatically produced the effort needed to implement it. Resources have not been made available in many countries. Moreover, the last few years have seen a frontal attack on the agenda's key feature, the holistic system approach. This attack has taken the shape of global initiatives in the health sector that have reintroduced the approach of addressing specific diseases and needs with little regard to the long-term impact on health systems. The sheer volume of global health initiatives has deflected policy and management attention from planning for integrative reproductive health programs.

Since 1994 activity and innovation in areas loosely classified as health sector reform have increased. Some reforms, especially those related to financing of health services, owe to recognition that the health sector is underfinanced because of low levels of tax-based public financing and the low budgetary priority typically given to health. Political forces beyond the health sector have initiated other reforms, such as decentralization. These reforms could have a strong impact on the way the health sector and reproductive health programs perform.

Further complicating matters are the new ways the donor community is managing and disbursing external support to low-income countries. A variety of financial instruments designed to strengthen systems and avoid difficulties in project financing have come onto the international health scene. They include

- the sectorwide approach, an attempt to integrate vertical programs and coordinate external donors;
- basket funding, a mechanism for harmonizing donor support;
- direct government budget support (rather than project financing); and
- poverty reduction strategy credits and programmatic lending/ credits, which take on multiple sectors' attempts to address structural issues that are barriers to poverty reduction.

Other new tools are medium-term expenditure frameworks, public expenditure–based credits, and public expenditure–based loans. Some of these tools have aggregated programs within the health sector, whereas others have been designed for reform of the entire economy of smaller countries.

Some in the reproductive health community are concerned about the impact of the reemergence of global health programs focused on individual health problems, new health sector reform initiatives, and new modes of external financial support. Are these changes attacks on the ICPD agenda, or are they opportunities for improving reproductive health? This book argues that the reproductive health community needs to better understand these changes to assess their impact on ICPD implementation and to develop the capacity and skills to take advantage of the changes and mitigate any negative impacts that they may already have produced. This chapter briefly explains these threats and opportunities and begins examination of the way forward.

## Reproductive Health and the Millennium Development Goals

During the 1990s, world leaders forged a consensus on agendas to improve human development during a series of global conferences that included the aforementioned 1994 International Conference on Population and Development in Cairo, the 1995 Conference on Women and Development in Beijing, and the 1995 Social Summit in Copenhagen. When the same leaders met five years later to assess progress in implementing these agendas, they agreed that there should be specific goals and indicators to measure results, so they proposed nine international development goals (IDGs), which included universal access to reproductive health information and services (an ICPD goal), improving gender equality, and reducing high rates of maternal and child mortality. When the same leaders assembled for the 2000 Millennium Summit and transformed the IDGs into the Millennium Development Goals (MDGs), they dropped reproductive health.

Exclusion of the reproductive health goal from the MDGs was a matter of political expediency (Girard 2001). Opponents of the goal had characterized it as promoting abortion and undermining family values by calling for sex education for adolescents. They threatened to block agreement on all the MDGs unless the reproductive health goal was eliminated. United Nations officials were under enormous pressure to have the Millennium Summit participants reach a consensus on the goals and relented to the demand of the few countries involved in the threat.

Because the MDGs play a prominent role in the setting of priorities by major donors, including the World Bank, the exclusion of reproductive health from the MDG list is a major challenge for the champions of reproductive health and rights. Funding for and attention to reproductive health could fall by the wayside unless a strong case can be made that failure to improve reproductive health and protect reproductive rights will undermine efforts to achieve other MDGs and reduce poverty. This theme was sounded in recent United Nations Population Fund State of World Population reports and in documents prepared for the Millennium Project.[1] One of the goals of chapters 9 (on expenditure tracking) and 12 (on priority setting) is to help reproductive health champions ensure that reproductive health and rights get adequate funding and attention as new approaches to resource allocation and program implementation are carried out under poverty reduction strategies and health system reform initiatives.

## Health Systems Are Failing Women, Especially Poor Women

In 1999 the World Bank reanalyzed 44 Demographic and Health Surveys (DHS), which are household surveys financed by the U.S. Agency for International Development, and calculated an asset index that allows identification of the relative wealth of households in terms of population-based quintiles (Gwatkin and others 2000). Researchers expected that in many countries the poor would be in worse shape than the better off with respect to health outcomes and health system outputs, but the depth and persistence of inequalities was much greater than they anticipated.

Inequalities were present in all measures of outcomes: infant and child mortality, maternal mortality, malnutrition, and fertility. Inequalities were also present in health system outputs across all forms of services, even those provided by the public sector without cost recovery. Most striking, services related to reproductive health were more inequitable than any other cluster of services (Gwatkin 2002).[2] In other words, the public health sectors designed to protect poor women are failing them in many parts of the developing world. (Chapter 8 presents an analysis of gender issues; chapter 9 presents an analysis of wealth-based inequality.)

The numbers illustrating this public system failure are depressingly consistent. Figure 1.1a shows the level of inequalities in attended deliveries in four South Asian countries in the early to mid-1990s. It reveals that the failure of the public sector to provide facility-based deliveries is almost complete and is greatest for the poorest women, less than 6 percent of who deliver at a public facility in the four countries. Data on antenatal (prenatal) care and medically attended delivery, regardless of location, show equally large public sector failures in the four countries.

***Figure 1.1*** *Attended Deliveries at Public Facilities: Poorest and Richest Quintiles*

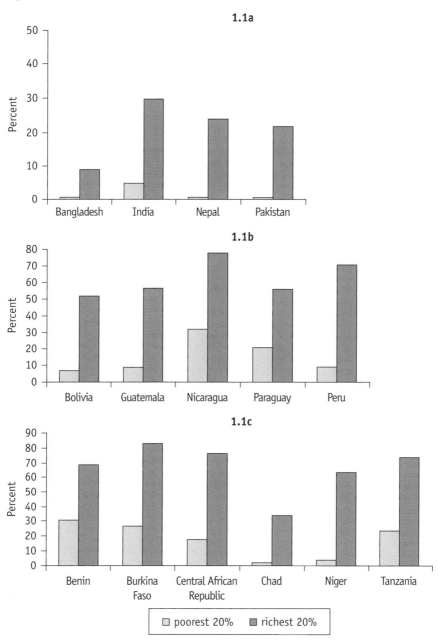

*Source:* Gwatkin and others 2000.

Public sector failure—both to make services physically available and to provide education and communication programs that increase demand for the services—is not unique to South Asia. Figure 1.1b highlights such failure in five Central and South American countries. Unlike the public health system in South Asia, that in Latin America appears to be doing a little better for the well-to-do in society: more than 50 percent of attended deliveries are deliveries by women in the richest quintile. But the gap between the rich and the poor is even bigger in Central and South America than in South Asia. A similar situation prevails in Sub-Saharan Africa. Figure 1.1c shows the levels of inequality in six countries in the region.

Absolute system failure may be a fair way of describing how badly public health care systems have performed in the area of reproductive health, especially for poor and vulnerable people. This failure has motivated the international health community to address the needs, if not the rights, of women around the world. The community's frustration with health systems' inability to deliver services to the most vulnerable is one reason for the large number of global health initiatives. Others have reacted to system failure by attempting to strengthen systems and by exploring new ways of making health sectors more responsive to needs. Yet others have reacted by attempting to change financial support modalities. They argue that fragmented support may have contributed to system failure and led governments to corrupt domestic budgeting mechanisms to please donors.

But the push to do something, whether create global initiatives or reform and strengthen systems, has been interpreted by many in the reproductive health community as a threat to implementation of the ICPD agenda. In September 2003 an international conference on the link between reproductive health and health system development at the University of Leeds exposed a sizable language and orientation gap between those advocating reproductive health and those focused on system reforms and strengthening. The main question that needs to be answered by those concerned about reproductive health objectives is whether system reforms and global initiatives are challenges to be overcome or opportunities to be exploited.

## Internal Threats to the Reproductive Health Agenda

Assessment of the challenges, opportunities, or both faced by the reproductive health community would be neither complete nor honest if it did not address the community's internal failures. Even in the absence of these failures, however, the environment of change described above may make implementation of the ICPD agenda across the globe difficult. If the agenda is to be realized anywhere, the international reproductive health community should focus its efforts on helping counterparts in individual countries in three areas: definition of the boundaries of reproductive health, advocacy, and empirical research.

### Definition of the Boundaries of Reproductive Health

Participants in the World Bank Institute's Reproductive Health and Health Sector Reform courses are asked to define the boundaries of reproductive health (see chapter 2 for an examination of these boundaries). They more often than not conclude that identifying the point at which reproductive health starts or stops is very difficult. This response is consistent with the holistic approach of the ICPD. But inability to clearly and convincingly define a program has a strongly negative impact on efforts to advocate for it when competing for public and donor resources.

The dilemma for people advocating for reproductive health is that to secure resources they have to simplify and streamline programs in ways that are counter to the inclusiveness of the ICPD agenda. It can be argued, however, that reproductive health is not an all-or-nothing situation and that the solution is for local communities and national programs to take a phased approach consistent with their financial and capacity constraints. In other words, it is conceivable to fashion a long-term vision of reproductive health that pushes boundaries and to define short- and medium-term programs that are manageable and relatively easy to sell to those who make decisions about budgets. Decisions about what should be given priority in the short and medium term have to take into account the needs of the country, and especially the needs of the poor and socially vulnerable.

### Advocacy

A refrain at the conference on reproductive health and health systems at the University of Leeds was that failure to follow a "rights-based" approach—an approach with appeal to many reproductive rights advocates and activists—is one reason for the failure of public systems to provide services to women. A more difficult question is to what extent this argument resonates with decision makers in countries where total public spending on health is in single-digit U.S. dollars per person per year. Given extreme financial and capacity constraints, the concept of rights may actually scare people away from opening doors they cannot control.  >

A more practical approach that might help the reproductive health community secure greater resources in low-income settings is to focus on expected outcomes and the extent to which investment in reproductive health services would save lives, reduce suffering, and help address socially and culturally challenging problems. The nutrition community took this approach in the early 1990s when it developed empirical bases for assessing the returns to investment in nutrition and produced a computer program that helps countries quantify outcomes in mortality, morbidity, loss of cognitive abilities in children, and loss of productivity in adults.[4] It is hard to argue against saying that all children should have the right to grow up free of hunger or nutritional deficiencies, but the argument that resonated in many poor countries was the focus on outcomes, not rights.

## Empirical Research

The reproductive health community (unlike the nutrition and child health communities) is not yet adept at measuring outcomes and has difficulty measuring the health system outputs needed to achieve outcomes and estimating the cost of interventions that produce outputs. In many ways, the reproductive health community has a wonderful story to tell, but it lacks the empirical foundation to make the story compelling to policy makers.

Maternal mortality and morbidity are among the reproductive health outcomes most often cited in arguing the benefit of investment in reproductive health, but in many countries these outcomes are not easy to measure consistently or over time. Nor is measuring health system outcomes in reproductive health easy. Take, for example, attended deliveries, which even in standardized surveys such as the DHS can be interpreted differently in different contexts, especially when comparing Africa and Asia. At issue are the delivery attendant's training, skills, and qualifications, which differ from region to region and country to country.

An even greater problem than the difficulty of measuring some health system outputs is the dearth of empirical evidence in the scientific literature on the types of health system outputs that can produce the desired reproductive health outcomes. Given difficulties in measuring outcomes and the system outputs needed to achieve them, and the lack of scientific clarity on how to achieve desired outcomes, it is not hard to see why policy and bud-get dialogue often fails to favor reproductive health services.

## A Way Forward

Much of the ambitious ICPD agenda has yet to be achieved. However, the reproductive health community's experience in attempting to implement it suggests practical steps for achieving much greater success by 2015. These steps include building local (in-the-field) capacity for advocacy efforts and marshalling empirical evidence and arguments to bolster these efforts.

### Capacity Building

Achieving tangible results will require sustained engagement by national representatives of the reproductive health community in every country that needs assistance. In other words, implementers of and activists for repro-ductive health programs need to be armed with the skills and tools required to engage in health sector reforms, to take advantage of global initiatives, and to effectively influence the new forms of aid support. These skills and tools include economics, finance, political mapping, epidemiology, and behavior change. Support for developing these skills and tools should be targeted to policy makers, managers, private sector contributors, civil soci-ety advocates, and academicians—the people who encounter the challenges and opportunities and who are the only ones that can do something about them at the national and subnational levels. In short, the reproductive health community in any given country should have the ability to

- empirically document reproductive health problems,
- diagnose the causes of the problems and identify obstacles to solving them,
- develop expenditure and other programs to implement new policies,
- influence the political decision-making process to help ensure that adopted policies are consistent with the reproductive health agenda and are likely to work,
- implement the reproductive health agenda, and
- monitor and evaluate performance to ensure that lessons are learned and applied.

Building capacity for such skills is not an easy or cheap exercise, but without them, the reproductive health community is likely to continue to stay on the outside trying to get in.

## A New Empiricism

While most reproductive health battles and engagement occur at national and subnational levels, much must be done at the global level to strengthen the hand of people on the front lines. For the reproductive health community to recapture the attention of policy makers and financiers, investments in quantification are needed. As noted above, the reproductive health community has difficulty measuring reproductive health outcomes; health system outputs likely to achieve these outcomes; and the cost and budgetary implications of designing, implementing, or expanding these health system outcomes. Without better command of empirical arguments, reproductive health advocates will find it difficult to convince decision makers that they have identified cost-effective programs that can be implemented within reasonable budget constraints. Investments in building empirical knowledge, evidence, and arguments are vital to the long-term success of the reproductive health agenda.

# 2

# *The Porous Boundaries of Reproductive Health*

Until 1994 reproductive health was thought of in terms of population policies and programs that focused principally on family planning aimed at slowing population growth. The International Conference on Population and Development (ICPD) held in Cairo that year changed this narrow focus by redefining reproductive health as a

> state of complete physical, mental and social well-being and not merely the absence of disease or infirmity, in all matters relating to the reproductive system and to its functions and processes. Reproductive health therefore implies that people are able to have a satisfying and safe sex life and that they have the capability to reproduce and the freedom to decide if, when and how often to do so. Implicit in this last condition are the rights of men and women to be informed and to have access to safe, effective, affordable and acceptable methods of family planning of their choice, as well as other methods for the regulation of fertility which are not against the law, and the right of access to appropriate health care services that will enable women to go safely through pregnancy and childbirth and provide couples the best chance of having a healthy infant. (United Nations 1995)

Thus the ICPD expanded reproductive health to address the full range of reproductive and sexual health needs of women and men. This major change was rooted in the human rights focus of the ICPD, according to which individuals and their needs should be given priority over demo-graphic imperatives. The ICPD also recognized changing demographic, epi-demiological, and programmatic realities.

The practical response to the policy reorientation demanded by the ICPD has been slow. The pace of this response is not surprising. Attitudes toward reproductive health have always been guarded. As noted in chapter 1, reproductive health was omitted from the Millennium Development Goals (MDGs) despite increasing awareness of the scope and importance of reproductive health problems. According to the United Nations Population Fund (UNFPA) *State of World Population 2005* report, several MDGs are dependent on improved reproductive health (UNFPA 2005).

In many countries, population programs have expanded access to contra-ceptives and lowered fertility, but progress is lacking in other major areas of reproductive health, notably maternal mortality and the prevention and management of sexually transmitted infections (STIs). With the steady wors-ening of the HIV/AIDS epidemic, neglect of this aspect of reproductive health has resulted in poor public health and is a violation of human rights.

## More than Health Care

In addressing the slow response to the ICPD agenda, reproductive health specialists have recognized that services that respect and respond to the needs of clients are more effective than those driven by top-down demo-graphic goals. Hence, informed clients who understand and choose a family planning method that suits them are more likely to continue using that method and are also more likely to utilize services that provide for their own and their families' needs.

While broadening the range of care to include "a constellation of meth-ods, techniques and services that contribute to reproductive health and well-being by preventing and solving health problems" (United Nations 1995), the ICPD definition also made it clear that reproductive health involves more than health care. It recognizes that poor reproductive health is often rooted in poverty and the subordination of women. Improvement in reproductive health outcomes—whether fewer unwanted pregnancies, reduced maternal and child mortality, or reduced incidence of STI—depends on contextual factors such as women's autonomy and empower-ment as well as the accessibility and quality of services.

Complications of pregnancy and delivery such as eclampsia, hemor-rhage, and obstructed labor are difficult to predict; all pregnant women are at risk of these conditions. Managing these risks requires effective antenatal care, skilled attendance at birth, and a functioning referral system. But availability of services is only one side of the equation; the other is affordability. Poor women are much less likely to have access to health care facilities or to be able to pay for care. They are therefore more likely to die or suffer adverse health consequences as a result of an emergency. Poor women are even more disadvantaged when gender systems are exclusionary. In many low-income settings, men may decide which members of the household will have access to health care. Gender imbalance lessens women's power to negotiate safe sex and increases risk when STIs and HIV/AIDS infection rates are high. >

<Reproductive health is not limited to the reproductive process or to reproductive ages. Poor nutrition for girls in childhood and adolescence is a major factor in poor reproductive outcomes for women and their children. Harmful practices such as female genital cutting, domestic violence, and sexual trafficking are detrimental to reproductive health and violate sexual and reproductive rights. And widely disparate factors, such as poorly managed obstetric emergencies and STIs, have adverse health consequences that extend beyond the reproductive age. >

The ICPD made gender equality, equity, and the empowerment of women high priorities. It also added sexual health and reproductive rights to established priorities such as safe motherhood, reproductive health, and high-quality family planning services. This broadening of the content and goals of reproductive health activities was imaginative, but it confused many administrations that were accustomed to packages of interventions and services managed by a single agency or ministry and that were coping with other fundamental economic and political changes. To be effective, the new focus required attention to the full range of factors that influence health outcomes—including attitudes, social cohesion, and health information—and to

- independent changes linked with structural adjustment, which in many cases led to the retreat of the state from the social sectors;
- decentralization of operating responsibilities—and, in some cases, fiscal and policy responsibilities—to the provincial or district level;
- development of a civil society, and nongovernmental organizations in particular, whose voice assumed a growing importance in reproductive health matters; and
- promotion of reproductive and sexual health by family planning programs that had formerly focused on simply preventing or spacing births.

## A New Way of Doing Business

The Program of Action drawn up at the ICPD presented an agenda of topics that had to be addressed in an integrated way. It implied a new way of working that is client-centered, rights-based, and gender-sensitive. And it introduced a role for groups hitherto neglected (such as young people, men, and refugees) and a concern for violence against women and female genital mutilation.

The Program of Action raised further challenges: how to measure, cost, and track changes. Establishing quantitative measures is often necessary to drive programs—as in the case of the under-five mortality rate and vaccine coverage rates that have given UNICEF's work momentum in recent years. To develop such measures requires clarity about the key factors that contribute to improvements in health. Until recently, such indicators have been lacking, because the models that describe reproductive health outcomes have been poorly articulated. Good measures for maternal mortality, a key indicator of the quality and coverage of obstetric services, exist, as do theory and empirical knowledge about how maternal deaths can be reduced. Thus indicators in this field are relatively easy to develop.

For other reproductive health outcome measures, the theory and evidence is diffuse. When dealing with gender relations and rights issues, the models and measures are even less well developed.[5] However, academics and practitioners are seeking to identify appropriate measures. We can think of at least four closely related dimensions of reproductive health:

- reproductive health status, as measured by indicators such as maternal mortality, infant mortality, and contraceptive prevalence;
- conditions associated with the reproductive organs and system;
- conditions exacerbated by sex and pregnancy; and
- social aspects of sex and reproduction.

To complicate matters, reproductive health is not just about numbers of deaths or illnesses: its social consequences are every bit as important as its medical outcomes. And its medical outcomes are often overlooked (for example: cumulative morbidity, comorbidity, and contraceptive morbidity, and conditions resulting from female genital mutilation[6]). Knowing the dimensions of the burden of reproductive ill health is insufficient. Other elements have to be taken into account, such as the proportion of the burden due to exposure to a specific risk, or the proportion that could be alleviated by reducing the risk, and how the risk might be mitigated.

A key risk factor for poor reproductive health is unsafe sex, a major subject of attention in reproductive health today. Unsafe sex leads to a catalogue of adverse consequences, including HIV/AIDS, STIs, unwanted pregnancy, unsafe abortion, and sexual violence. In generalized HIV epidemics, most HIV infections are attributable to unsafe sex; in 2000 some 3.3 million deaths (6 percent of total) were attributable to unsafe sex.

Addressing HIV/AIDS means addressing risks and vulnerabilities related to sexual behaviors. Consequently, the reproductive health community has had to influence and support behavior change aimed at safer sex, adolescent health, male involvement, community awareness, family planning needs of HIV-positive women, and prevention of mother-to-child disease transmission, as well as voluntary confidential counseling and testing, detection, and management of STIs.

Reproductive health has thus become multidimensional; its policies and interventions now extend beyond health *per se*. To complicate further the problems of definition and measurement, changes in the scope and nature of reproductive health interventions are taking place within the broader context of health sector reform.

# 3

# A Moving Target: Demographic and Epidemiological Changes

Planning for reproductive and other health services needs to reflect changing demographic and epidemiological conditions. This chapter discusses what is known as the demographic transition and considers the implications of demographic and epidemiological shifts for health systems, economic growth, and poverty reduction.

## Changing Demographics: The Demographic Transition

The second half of the 20th century was a period of major demographic changes. Global population in 1950 was approximately 2.5 billion. By the end of the century, it was over 6 billion (see figure 3.1). Almost all (more than 90 percent) of the increase in population took place in the world's demographic "south"—countries in Asia, Africa, and Latin America. The population of countries in the demographic "north" (Europe, North America, Japan, and Oceania) grew much more slowly.[7] One effect of this differential increase in population size was that the demographic balance between north and south of the 20th century had shifted much more to the south compared to what it had been at the beginning of the century. Compared with overall population increase, growth in urban population globally was even more rapid, particularly in the south.

Driving these changes is a process that demographers label the *demographic transition,* which is a way of describing how changing birth and

**Figure 3.1** *Demographic Transition, 1850–2050*

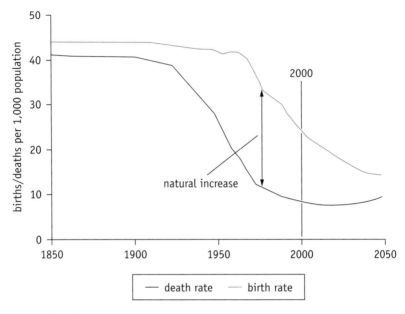

Source: United Nations 1998.

death rates, along with migration, brought about the large increases in human population size that began in the demographic north around the time of the Industrial Revolution and then accelerated when countries in the demographic south started to experience demographic transitions after World War II. For most of human history, birth and death rates were typically high and sometimes fluctuated as a result of upswings in mortality caused by disease outbreaks, famines, and wars.

Demographic transitions began when improvements in living conditions and public health decreased the frequency and severity of catastrophic mortality and eventually led to sustained mortality decline. Birth rates generally decline later than death rates, so that the rate of natural increase (the difference between birth and death rates) increases temporarily during the middle stages of the transition. When declines in birth rates catch up with death rates, natural increase also declines. Eventually birth and death rates reach low levels, though still subject to fluctuations such as the baby booms experienced by many northern countries after World War II and upswings in mortality associated with wars and disease outbreaks. Figure 3.2 depicts the demographic transition—though without migration and the fluctuations just mentioned.

**Figure 3.2** *Population Growth Trends, 1750–2150*

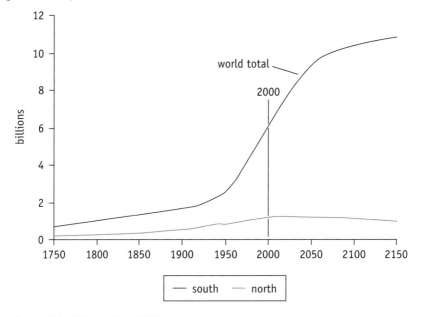

Source: United Nations 1996, 1998.

Countries in the demographic north went through their demographic transitions during the late 19th and early 20th centuries. The demographic south, with the exception of a couple of Latin American countries, began its transitions just after World War II. Improvements in medical technology (including antibiotics) accelerated mortality decline in southern countries, so that their increases in natural increase were much steeper than those that the north experienced early. Furthermore, emigration from Europe during its demographic transition dampened the impact of rising natural increase on European population growth (and increased the rate of growth in receiving countries in North and South America and in Oceania). Population growth rates, which had ranged between 1 and 2 percent per year during the northern transition, often reached 3 to 4 percent in the south.

## Impacts of Demographic Transitions

Concerns about the potentially adverse impact of rapid population increase on economic growth in the south prompted many countries and donor agencies to promote family planning in order to slow population growth rates. New contraceptive technologies (for example, the birth control pill) were being introduced at the time and were viewed as a way to balance the impact of the medical advances that had accelerated mortality decline. Experts debate the extent to which interventions such as organized family planning hastened fertility declines in the south relative to social and economic changes (for example, increased educational and employment opportunities for women), which played a more prominent role in fertility declines in northern countries. Whatever the cause, recent fertility declines in the south have been more rapid than those that occurred earlier in the north. Even with the recent slowdown of population growth rates in the south, the higher growth rates that prevailed during the decades when mortality declined more rapidly than fertility helped to double the size of population in the demographic south between 1950 and 2000.

Another feature of demographic changes during the last half of the 20th century was the varying pace of change among regions in the south. The transition occurred earlier and more rapidly in Latin America and East Asia than in South Asia and the Middle East. The transition has advanced least in Africa, as can be seen in figure 3.3, which shows regional trends in the total fertility rate (the number of births a woman has during her reproductive years).

**Figure 3.3** *Fertility Trends in Different Regions, 1950–2050*

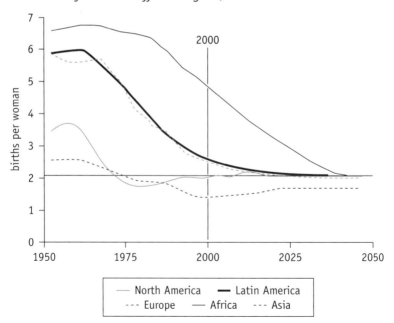

*Source:* United Nations 1998.

Fertility rates in North America and Europe are now lower than two births per woman (they rose briefly during the post-World War II baby booms in those regions). Fertility rates in Latin America and Asia dropped from around six in the 1950s to below three in 2000 and continue to decrease. Fertility decline is just getting started in Africa, and rates remain at pretransition levels in many countries (for example, Niger and Uganda).

Regional differences in mortality are another feature of the changing demographic landscape, as can be seen in figure 3.4, which shows regional trends in life expectancy—the average number of years that individuals in a population can expect to live given existing mortality rates. Life expectancy in North America and Europe already exceeds 70, and Latin America and Asia are approaching that level. Life expectancy in Africa was rising during the 1960s and 1970s but leveled off (and in many countries actually declined) as a result of the HIV/AIDS epidemic.

The long-term demographic impact of HIV/AIDS remains an uncertainty (not only for Africa, but also for China, India, and Russia, which have incipient epidemics). Demographers have studied the effects of the epidemic on birth and death rates in affected areas and found that HIV/AIDS

**Figure 3.4** *Regional Trends in Life Expectancy, 1925–2050*

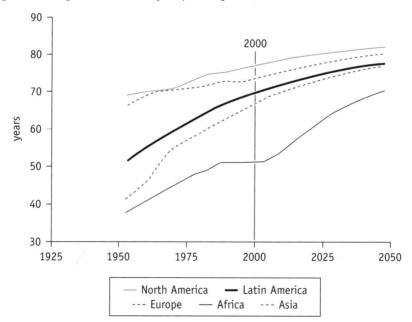

*Source:* United Nations 1998.

reduces fertility as well as increases mortality. The demographic effects can be severe in high-prevalence areas, though the effect on overall population increase is less than the adverse social and economic impacts of the disease (Epstein 2004).

One reason is that the interval between the time individuals become infected (for women, typically ages 15–24) and the time they die may be a decade or more (depending on a variety of factors, including the availability of treatment). Many HIV-positive women bear children (some of them HIV–positive) before they die, leaving AIDS orphans to be cared for by surviving relatives or in many cases to live on their own. The HIV/AIDS epidemic has forced demographers to rethink their assumption that mortality decline, once under way, was an unstoppable process. Reversals may also occur as the result of resurgent diseases like tuberculosis, malaria, and avian flu.

## Demographics of Age Composition

Another important dimension of global and regional shifts in population size and the forces that drive them are changes in the age composition of populations. High fertility in predemographic-transition societies creates a youthful age distribution in which a high proportion of the population is under age 15. As mortality and fertility rates decline, the age composition changes. Figure 3.5 shows the age distribution of the populations of three countries using what demographers call population age pyramids. Pyramids show the population in five-year age groups, starting with ages 0–4. The age pyramid for the Democratic Republic of Congo is typical of high-fertility countries, where more than half of the population is age 20 or younger. At the other extreme is Germany, whose population is experiencing negative growth because death rates are higher than birth rates. The shift from a broad-based youthful age structure to a top-heavy older age structure has important implications for national economies and budgets, particularly for pensions and health care.

## Epidemiological Transitions

Accompanying these shifts in age compositions are *epidemiological transitions*, or changes in the prevalence of the diseases that cause deaths. In high-mortality countries, most deaths are caused by infectious diseases (respiratory infections, diarrhea, malaria, and so on), and a large proportion of those dying are children. As medicines, public health, and improved living conditions helped control infections and reduced child mortality, people

**Figure 3.5**  *Population Pyramids of Three Countries*

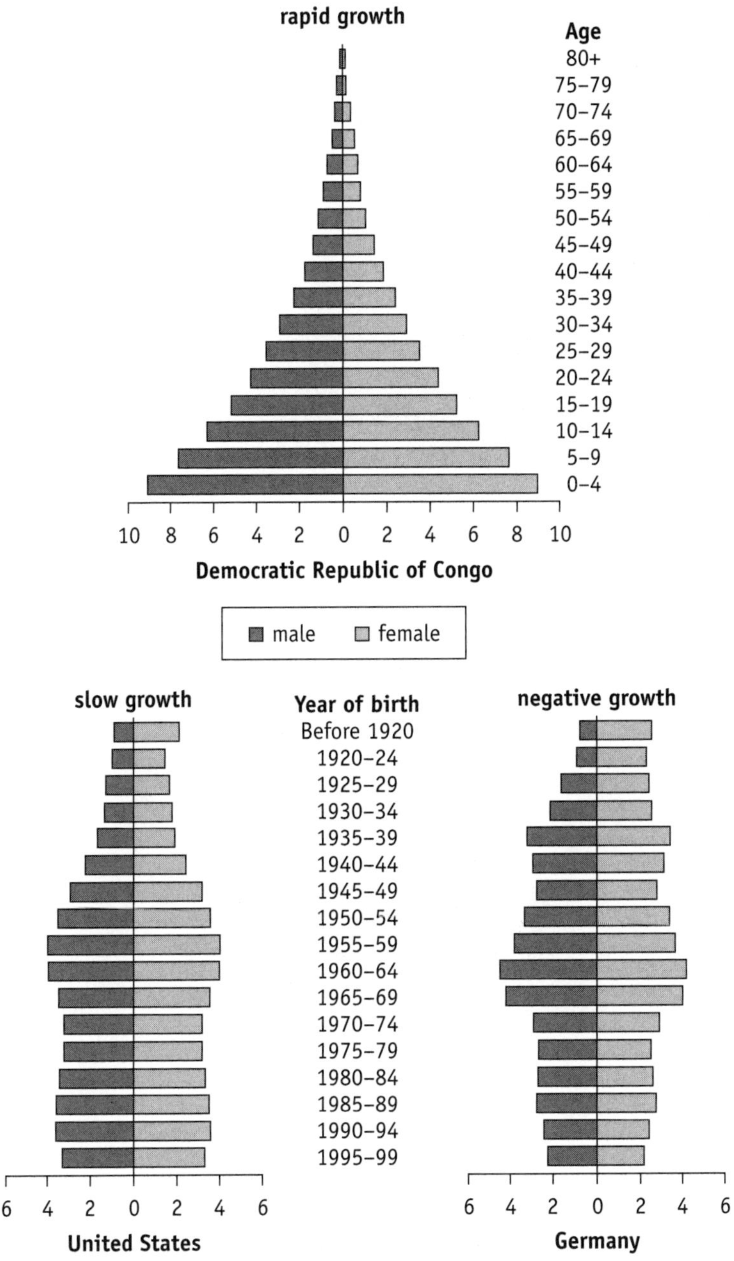

**rapid growth**

| Age |
|---|
| 80+ |
| 75–79 |
| 70–74 |
| 65–69 |
| 60–64 |
| 55–59 |
| 50–54 |
| 45–49 |
| 40–44 |
| 35–39 |
| 30–34 |
| 25–29 |
| 20–24 |
| 15–19 |
| 10–14 |
| 5–9 |
| 0–4 |

10  8  6  4  2  0  2  4  6  8  10

**Democratic Republic of Congo**

■ male    □ female

**slow growth**   **Year of birth**   **negative growth**

Before 1920
1920–24
1925–29
1930–34
1935–39
1940–44
1945–49
1950–54
1955–59
1960–64
1965–69
1970–74
1975–79
1980–84
1985–89
1990–94
1995–99

6  4  2  0  2  4  6          6  4  2  0  2  4  6

**United States**                     **Germany**

*Source:* United Nations 1998.

began to live longer, and the proportion of deaths attributable to other causes (accidents, violence, and noncommunicable diseases) rose. These epidemiological shifts are reflected in figure 3.6, which shows the distribution of the leading causes of death in Africa and Europe in 1998.

**Figure 3.6**  *Leading Causes of Death in Africa and Europe, 1998*

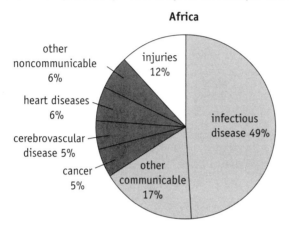

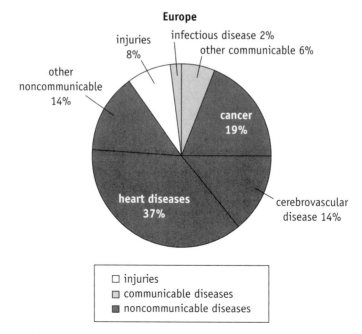

*Source:* WHO 1999, Ratzan, Filerman, and Lesar 2000.

In Africa, communicable diseases account for two-thirds of all deaths, while cancers, circulatory, and other noncommunicable diseases account for less than a quarter of deaths. In Europe, the picture is reversed. Communicable diseases account for less than 10 percent of deaths, while cancers, circulatory, and noncommunicable diseases account for more than four-fifths of deaths.

Health systems in countries that are in the early stages of their demographic and epidemiological transitions tend to focus on infant and child mortality and the infections that cause them, along with maternal conditions associated with high fertility, whereas health systems in countries at the other end of the epidemiological and demographic transition process deal with diseases that affect older populations. The transition process puts special stress on health systems and the economies that have to pay for them. For countries experiencing transitions, the shifts do not occur evenly within their populations. Richer and more urbanized segments of their population typically enjoy earlier gains than the poorer and rural segments. Because urban elites often have greater influence over national spending priorities, they may divert resources toward their health needs at the expense of the rural poor.

Countries that are more advanced in their demographic and epidemiological transitions face other challenges. One key difference between communicable and noncommunicable diseases is that the proportion of people who contract and then die from a communicable disease is higher than the proportion affected by noncommunicable diseases. In the latter case, people may survive a long time and require ongoing treatment (with its attendant demands on the health system) to survive. Because these people are also older and not working, health systems that depend on contributions from the working-age population to support pensions and health care for their elderly will also experience fiscal stress as the proportion of workers falls and the proportion of the elderly increases (for example, in Germany, which has a rapidly aging population and a wage-tax-based social insurance system).

## Implications of Demographic and Epidemiological Shifts

These issues underline age composition as the key link between demographic and epidemiological shifts, on the one hand, and national economics and budgets, on the other. Feedbacks from altered age composition work through many channels, the strength and direction of which depend on the pace at which changes (declines in birth and death rates and corresponding age shifts) occur. As figure 3.7 shows, countries do not move immediately from Congo-like age pyramids to the Germany-like pyramid shown in figure 3.5. Instead, the shift in age composition occurs in a wave-like manner; the crest of the wave moves first across the young adult population and then across the middle and finally the older ages as declining fertility and mortality take effect. The wave's speed and impact (shown in the bulge in the young adult group in figure 3.7) depend on how high birth (and to a lesser extent, death) rates were before the transition and on how rapidly they fall.

In figure 3.7, the red bars represent the age distribution of a pretransition population and the green bars, the posttransition situation. The solid red line, which peaks with a bulge centered in the 20–24 age group (or cohort), is the distribution that one might find in a population that is moving rapidly through the transition from high to low fertility and mortality. The proportion of population under age 15 has declined because of lower birth rates, but the proportion of population at older ages has not yet had a chance to increase (though it will when the bulge cohort gets older).

One feedback from these age shifts is demographic momentum. The young adult population is also the reproductive-age population. Depending on how large this population is relative to other cohorts, it can cause substantial absolute increases in population even when fertility is declining. For example, if the fertility rate has declined from six to three births per woman

**Figure 3.7** *Age Structure Profile*

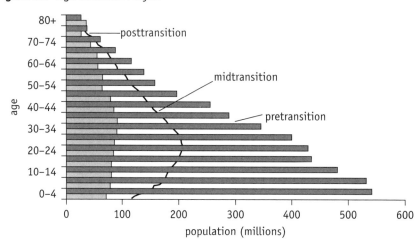

*Source:* United Nations 1998.

but the reproductive-age population has more than doubled during the interval that fertility rates declined, there will be *more* births during the transition than there were when it got started (mortality shifts also play a role in demographic momentum, though not as significant a one as fertility).

Demographers refer to this phenomenon as *demographic momentum*. Demographic momentum is a key reason why population size will continue to grow in the demographic south well into the 21st century. Momentum will account for half or more of the population increase in Asian and Latin American countries that have experienced rapid fertility declines but continued increases in absolute size.

Demographic momentum raises additional challenges for population policy. Once family planning programs have succeeded in lowering fertility rates, there may be a tendency to consider the "population problem" solved. In fact, the need for family planning is even greater because of the large number of women at reproductive age and their need to sustain fertility regulation. But fertility regulation alone is not enough. Demographic momentum is affected by the time interval between generations, which is related to the age of marriage and the initiation of childbearing. To the extent that the initiation of childbearing may be delayed by provision of alternatives to childbearing through increased education and economic opportunity, some of the momentum effect can be reduced. Social policy that reduces gender inequalities is worth pursuing in its own right, but it also has important demographic benefits that offset demographic momentum and help to reduce fertility rates.

Other feedbacks of changing age composition are those that can affect economic growth through savings and consumption patterns. In the early stages of the demographic transitions in the south, demographers and economists speculated that the high ratio of children to workers in those settings (demographers call it the *child-dependency ratio*) would divert resources from savings/investment to increase the productive potential of economies. For a variety of reasons (one that unequal income distributions could have dampened the impact of household consumption on national savings and investment), the adverse effect of child dependency did not turn out to be as important as expected, though concerns about it stimulated spending on national family planning programs.

As already noted, *old-age dependency* (the rising ratio of pensioners to workers) raises substantial concerns in countries that have pay-as-you-go financing for social insurance. The capacity of societies to address this problem depends on how dependent countries are on current tax revenues and on the strength of the economies that generate those revenues. Aging populations have prompted many governments to reexamine the ways in which they pay for the health and retirement benefits of their elderly. These concerns have also prompted researchers to revisit the question of how changes in age composition affect savings, investment, and economic growth during other stages of the demographic transition—for example, the middle stages when countries experience the demographic bulge in their population of young adults. This bulge contributes to demographic momentum, because these adults are at peak childbearing age.

Recent research suggests that some countries in East Asia (Taiwan, China; the Republic of Korea) experienced a "demographic bonus" as a result of the bulge that occurred in their working-age populations when they were a decade or two into their rapid demographic transitions. Bloom and others (2004) analyzed trend data on population and economic growth in East Asia for the 1980s and early 1990s and found that fertility decline and associated changes in the age structure of populations created demographic windows of opportunity in Taiwan and Korea. When combined with good economic policies (investments in human capital, production of goods that required the skills in which those investments were made, openness to trade, and good governance), the favorable age distribution produced a demographic bonus that would not have occurred without rapid fertility decline. This approach is more nuanced than earlier population growth analysis in that it examines both the positive and negative impact of population on growth and focuses on different phases of the demographic transition. Analysts have also been quick to point out that the "bonus" is both dependent on good economic policies and temporary (it comes after child dependency declines and before old-age dependency takes over, which can be very soon in rapidly aging populations) (Birdsall and others 2001).

Some economists are skeptical about the applicability of the demographic bonus argument outside East Asia, and even about its contribution to savings in East Asia (Ahlburg 2002; Schultz 2004). For example, Schultz replicated estimates of the impact of favorable demographics in East Asia on savings and found that the impact was reduced substantially when one of the variables (lagged savings) was made endogenous. Indeed, some economists voice concern that inappropriate economic and social policies (such as failure to educate women and involve them in productive activities) may keep South Asian countries now experiencing rapid demographic changes from enjoying the benefits that their East Asian neighbors were able to reap. Assessments of Latin America's demographics over the past two to three decades suggest that economic inequality may have under-mined the capacity of many countries in that region to benefit fully from their rapid demographic transitions.

Additional country-level studies are needed to address these issues and to show what could be done to enhance the demographic bonus potential in countries that do not have the institutional and organizational advantages enjoyed by the East Asian countries when they experienced it. More atten-tion also needs to be given to whether and how bonus-driven economic growth can be translated into improved living standards for poor people within countries enjoying a demographic bonus. One would hope that macro-level links among fertility, age structure, and capital formation would reflect or be consistent with changes in household-level demograph-ics and the prospects of individuals and households to escape poverty.

Demography is not destiny, but public policies that fail to take account of the role that demography plays in demand for public services like health, education, and social services, and in the capacity to mobilize the resources to provide such services, can find themselves blindsided by the conse-quences of demographic change. Fortunately, the target moves slowly, but failure to recognize and react appropriately to demographic changes can take a long time to correct and be much more difficult to fix.

# 4

# The Alphabet Soup of International Development Aid

As noted in chapter 1, one of the challenges faced by the health sector and the reproductive health community relates to the changing financial architecture of development assistance. On one hand, frustrations with failures in many health systems have led to a seemingly never-ending list of global health initiatives that seek to achieve positive health outcomes in spite of weak health systems. On the other hand, frustrations with verticality and efforts to bypass health systems have led donors (many of which support vertical initiatives) to promote attempts to work programmatically not only within sectors but across them.

As a result of these two trends in financial support mechanisms, the reproductive health community finds itself pulled in opposite directions: vertical initiatives and multisector programs. This chapter examines this state of affairs and the main players in international development assistance.

## Serial Global Initiatives: Too Much of a Good Thing!

A clear threat to any broad approach to improving health systems is a return to vertical approaches and competing disease-driven agendas. The International Conference on Population and Development (ICPD) agenda is clearly under threat from the amazing growth in global health initiatives, which individually are extremely well meaning but as a totality threaten any attempt at rational support to the world's neediest countries, especially where health systems are weak. A Google.com search for "global health initiative" resulted in the following list, which is in no particular order and which would have been longer had the search extended beyond 15 minutes:

- Women's Health Initiative
- WHO–UNAIDS HIV Vaccine Initiative
- WHO's 3 by 5 Initiative
- Global Alliance for Vaccines and Immunizations
- Global Polio Eradication Initiative
- UN Global Media AIDS Initiative
- Tobacco Control Global Initiative
- Global Health Information Network
- Roll Back Malaria
- Reproductive Health Initiative International Project
- Red Cross and Red Crescent ARCHCI Africa Health Initiative
- New Global Initiative to Combat Interpersonal Violence
- The Nation's Voice on Mental Illness Global Partnership Initiative
- Measles Initiative
- Malaria Vaccine Initiative
- Global Initiative for Asthma Learning Program
- International AIDS Vaccine Initiative
- IMB's Global Health Care Initiative
- Global Health Trust
- The Hope Initiative
- Stop TB
- The Global TB Research Initiative
- Global School Health Initiative
- Global Initiative to Strengthen Maternal and Reproductive Health Services
- Global Initiative to Fight Hunger
- Global Initiative for the Elimination of Avoidable Blindness
- Global Health Equity Initiative
- Global Health Action
- Global Initiative to Educate Women about Contraception
- Diabetes Action Now
- Canadian International Immunization Initiative
- Integrated Management of Childhood Illnesses
- The Breast Health Global Initiative for Countries with Limited Resources
- Global Initiative to Promote the Consumption of Fruits and Vegetables

Taken individually, many of these initiatives make a lot of sense. Materials on the initiatives' Web sites reflect the sense of urgency and frustration with health system failures. They highlight the basic dilemma of either acting quickly to address a pressing health need or thinking holistically and systematically about reforming and improving the health sector. The solution is probably to take quick action on some health outcomes but on most to effect systemic change. The balancing point probably differs from country to country and depends on both the nature of the health needs and the extent of system capacity and failure.

Regardless of the correct balance between short-term action and long-term system investment, the current environment of serial global initiatives may be complicating the picture for many low-income and low-capacity countries—especially when their governments must spend limited human resources on filling out applications, maintaining parallel information systems, producing specific reports, and demonstrating ownership of globally designed vertical initiatives in order to get funding. These initiatives typically divert the attention of client countries' most qualified individuals from managing health systems to attending to the initiatives' information needs. Moreover, the initiatives pose a direct threat to reproductive health issues and programs at the country level, because they favor activities that are easy to define and relatively easy to implement in narrow and vertical ways. By doing so, they undermine the broad approach advocated at the ICPD in Cairo.

At the global level, serial global initiatives, especially large initiatives focused on communicable diseases, pose a different threat to the reproductive health agenda. This threat is manifested in the competition for attention and resources from donor countries and technical and financial agencies. Because human and financial resources for development assistance are limited, the new and large initiatives can be expected to receive the lion's share. Consequently, the reproductive health community is left to fight for attention and resources to reinvigorate support for the ICPD agenda. This struggle will force the reproductive health community to find ways to simplify and make operational the program of work, as well as to become much more adept at quantifying expected outcomes, the outputs needed to achieve those outcomes, and the resources and inputs needed to produce the outputs. The ability to make the argument for resources and to measure results and effectiveness is critical in this development aid environment.

The new global initiatives do sometimes offer opportunities for those interested in furthering the reproductive health agenda. We should not simply dismiss all these initiatives as too vertical and fail to take advantage of opportunities to help countries to get badly needed resources for programs that fall within reproductive health. Consider, for example, how resources for HIV/AIDS can be used to strengthen reproductive health services in Africa and Asia.

## From Projects to Sectorwide Approaches to Budget Support Programs

Some experts are urging donors and lenders to move away from the verticality and project focus of the proliferating global initiatives and instead look to sectorwide approaches and budget support programs. In some ways, this push away from projects is another reaction to wide system failure.

The argument for changing how donors and lenders support governments reflects frustration with approaches focused on simple and measurable outcomes in the short run rather than on the critical functions of local institutions and on the importance of addressing systemic weaknesses. This argument, by no means new, was reinvigorated by *World Development Report 2004: Making Services Work for Poor People,* and is dominating the development assistance debate within international financial institutions and many bilateral donors.

The argument is that a fragmented approach to aid flows has a strongly negative impact on service delivery and priority-setting mechanisms in recipient countries. In addition, this approach results in high transaction costs due to the many parallel structures developed and maintained to address the needs of the donor/lender. Another negative impact of the vertical or project approach is that donors/lenders select the inputs they want to provide (on the basis of either what they deem important or how their aid is tied to the goods and services they are providing), leaving the domestic budget to cover other expenditures and by doing so creating a two-sided dependency.

It can be argued that a donor-coordinated, sectorwide approach that is aligned to the recipients' budgeting and institutional setup is much more effective than a project-based or vertical approach to supporting the health sector in the long run, because it helps countries develop local systems that remain after aid ends. An even more holistic aid approach would be a budget support modality that goes beyond one sector and allows countries to receive aid directly into their budget in an untied fashion but against agreed expenditure plans and expected outcomes.

This relatively new way of doing business offers opportunities as well as risks for the reproductive health community. At issue is the extent to which reproductive health activities receive more or less attention and resources in a project versus a program approach to financial aid. More specifically, an empirical question is the extent to which the health sector gets more or less money from national budgets and then the extent to which reproductive health programs receive more or less money. The answer, again, is that it depends on the ability of the reproductive health community to support client countries, and especially the individuals and groups looking after the reproductive health function in these countries.

For reproductive health concerns to be addressed in a sectorwide or programmatic approach, an empirically convincing case needs to be made to decision makers within client countries' ministries of health and finance as well as to donors and lenders supporting health programs. Such a case needs to be made with recognition that resources will be insufficient to do everything. Thus, strategic thinking is needed to phase in support.

## ⟨ Alphabet Soup

A by-product of the complexity of the financial and technical architecture of aid in the health sector is a seemingly endless list of acronyms. A detailed explanation of the functions of the agencies, global initiatives, and financial instruments represented by these acronyms is beyond the scope of this book, but the glossaries below may be helpful to those in the reproductive health community who are working at the national level.

### Multilateral Agencies

Let us start with international finance organizations/institutions, also known as IFIs:

- The World Bank (occasionally referred to as the Bank, a designation not appreciated by the other development banks) consists of four groups: IDA, IBRD, IFC, and MIGA.

  - IDA: The International Development Agency serves low-income World Bank clients (the World Bank classifies low-income countries on the basis of the level of their gross domestic products per capita). The most obvious difference between IDA and IBRD (see next bullet) is that low-income countries served by IDA can borrow at a highly discounted interest rate with long maturity time frames.

- IBRD: The International Bank for Reconstruction and Development serves middle-income country clients through lending and nonlending products.
- IFC: The International Finance Cooperation is the only group within the World Bank that works with nongovernmental entities. It works directly with the private sector.
- MIGA: The Multilateral Investment Guarantee Agency insures investments in order to promote foreign direct investments in emerging economies.

- IMF: The International Monitory Fund is the sister organization of the World Bank. It focuses on client countries' macroeconomic stability and fiscal and monetary policy.
- IDB: The Inter-American Development Bank is the development bank that serves the Americas region.
- ADB: The Asian Development Bank is the development bank that serves large parts of Asia.
- AfDB: The African Development Bank is the development bank that serves Africa.

Multilateral technical agencies (MTAs):

- WHO: The World Health Organization is the United Nations specialized agency for health. Supporting WHO in this task are six regional offices.

  - AFRO covers most of Africa.
  - EMRO covers the Eastern Mediterranean region.
  - EURO covers Europe and Central Asia.
  - PAHO covers the Americas.
  - SEARO covers South and East Asia.
  - WPRO covers the Western Pacific region.

- UNFPA: United Nations Population Fund
- UNICEF: United Nations Children's Fund
- UNDP: United Nations Development Programme

Although these IFIs and MTAs are governed by the same countries, each groups countries in a different way. For example, the World Bank and WHO place different countries in their regional groups, making it a little harder for the two agencies to work together. The EMRO regional office includes countries classified in three different World Bank regions (Africa, the Middle East, and South Asia).

## Bilateral Agencies

Many high-income countries have governmental agencies that provide financial, and occasionally technical, assistance to low- and low-middle income countries. Some countries, such as Germany, have more than one agency providing development assistance. Bilateral agencies, with a few exceptions such as the Netherlands, are known by their acronyms: Australia (AUSAID), Canada (CIDA), United Kingdom (DfID, previously ODA), Germany (GTZ and KfW), Japan (JICA), Norway (NORAD), Sweden (SIDA), and the USA (USAID).

## Foundations

Foundations have always had an impact on the general direction of health sector strategies and reforms in developing countries, but the last few years have seen a major shift in foundations' power, thanks mainly to the entry of the Bill and Melinda Gates Foundation into the aid picture. Because this foundation can bring substantial amounts of money to the table and has the flexibility to use this money without restrictions, it can focus on neglected areas and bring heft to major new initiatives. Other foundations continue to bring a technical and issues focus to health matters and, in some cases, to reproductive health. These foundations include the William and Flora Hewlett Foundation, the David and Lucile Packard Foundation, and the Rockefeller Foundation.

## Global Health Initiatives

The Google search discussed above evidences the growth of initiatives. A recently completed review of the largest global health initiatives (Granstrom and Yazbeck 2006) identified 22 global initiatives focusing on a combination of objectives: advocacy, funding, research and development, and technical assistance. The review resulted in a two-page fact sheet on each of these initiatives, listed here in alphabetical order:

- AHPSR: Alliance for Health Policy and Systems Research
- DNDi: Drugs for Neglected Diseases initiative
- FIND: Foundation for Innovative New Diagnostics (of the European Observatory on Health Systems and Policies)
- GAIN: Global Alliance for Improved Nutrition
- GAVI: Global Alliance for Vaccines and Immunization
- GDF: Global TB Drug Facility

- GFATM: Global Fund to Fight AIDS, Tuberculosis and Malaria
- HRP: UNDP/UNFPA/WHO/World Bank Special Program of Research, Development and Research Training in Human Reproduction
- IAVI: International AIDS Vaccine Initiative
- INDEPTH: International Network of field sites with continuous Demographic Evaluation of Populations and Their Health in developing countries
- ITI: International Trachoma Initiative
- MIM: Multinational Initiative on Malaria
- MMV: Medicines for Malaria Venture
- PCD: Partnership for Child Development
- RBM: Roll Back Malaria Partnership
- Safe Motherhood: Partnership for Safe Motherhood and Newborn Health
- TB Alliance: TB Partnership, Global Alliance for TB Drug Development
- TDR: UNICEF/UNDP/World Bank/WHO Special Program for Research and Training in Tropical Diseases
- UNAIDS: Joint United Nations Programme on HIV/AIDS  >

# 5

## HIV/AIDS and Reproductive Health: Competitors or Natural Allies?

The 1994 International Conference on Population and Development (ICPD) extended the boundaries of reproductive health, but HIV/AIDS has wrought the greatest change in how family planning and maternal and child health are viewed. The HIV/AIDS epidemic has had a devastating impact on people throughout the world. In 2003, about 14,000 people were infected with HIV each day (5.1 million per year); of these people, almost 2,000 (730,000 per year) were children under 15 years of age, and about 12,000 (4.4 million per year) were persons aged 15 to 49 years. Fifty percent of the newly infected within the 15–49 age group were women,[8] and 50 percent of these women were 15 to 24 years old. In 2003, some 17 million women were living with HIV/AIDS, and some 2.3 million births were to HIV-positive women.

Three of the Millennium Development Goals (MDGs) relate directly to reproductive health and HIV/AIDS:

- Goal 4: Reduce child mortality
- Goal 5: Improve maternal health
- Goal 6: Combat HIV/AIDS, malaria, and other diseases

It can be argued that Goal 3 (promote gender equality and empower women) is a fundamental principle for achieving good reproductive health and that Goal 2 (achieve universal primary education) is necessary to direct more health education messages to more people in the reproductive age population and that women with higher educational levels have smaller desired and actual family sizes. In one way or another, all the MDGs are affected by HIV/AIDS. As Kofi Annan expressed it: "All the development gains of the past decades are being eroded by HIV/AIDS." Attainment of the MDGs is therefore impossible without tackling this cross-cutting issue.

Understanding how to maximize the synergies between reproductive health on the one hand and HIV/AIDS policy, programming, and services on the other will help governments, NGOs, and donors identify better working and funding mechanisms. In particular, it will have a positive impact on donors' commitment to scaling up basic services, harmonizing support of country programs, and strengthening health systems, as well as on sectorwide approaches, general budget support, global partnerships, and so on. Knowing how to promote synergies at country, regional, and international levels is therefore critical to achieving universal access to basic services and meeting MDG targets.

## Effects of HIV/AIDS on Reproductive Health

Data on HIV/AIDS are alarming and widely publicized, but information about the effects of HIV on reproductive health is not so widely disseminated and understood. For women who are HIV positive, pregnancy and delivery complications may be more severe, and miscarriages and stillbirths are more common. Risk of cervical and other genital cancers is also increased. For both men and women with HIV, tuberculosis, anemia, and malaria can be worse, and sexually transmitted infections (STIs) can be more severe and difficult to treat. Men too suffer the increased risk of genital cancer.

According to Askew and Berer (2003), "approximately 80 percent of HIV cases are transmitted sexually and a further 10 percent, perinatally or during breastfeeding. Hence, the health sector has looked to sexual and reproductive health programs for leadership and guidance in providing information and counseling to prevent these forms of transmission, and more recently to undertake some aspects of treatment."

As the AIDS epidemic matures, new challenges for both HIV prevention and reproductive health service delivery are emerging. First, as AIDS treatment programs expand, there are new opportunities for HIV prevention, including reproductive health services for positive people and those vulnerable to HIV infection. What circumstances are necessary to maximize these opportunities and limit the risk of an emerging drug-resistant HIV epidemic? Second, in some countries with a high HIV prevalence, maternal mortality ratios are reported to have increased dramatically. What constrains the effective integration of evidence-based and appropriate HIV prevention and care interventions within maternity services?

Over the past decade considerable work has been undertaken (for example, by the Population Council and the London School of Hygiene and Tropical Medicine) to explore and test ways of integrating HIV/AIDS and reproductive health information and service delivery. More recently there have been many declarations of support for strengthening links between HIV/AIDS and reproductive health work. For example, in May 2004 the Glion Call to Action on Family Planning and HIV/AIDS in Women and Children was signed by UN agencies, donors, and civil society. In June 2004, UNFPA and UNAIDS, together with ministers, parliamentarians, ambassadors, leaders of other UN organizations, government officials, and civil society representatives, signed the New York Call to Commitment—Linking HIV/AIDS and sexual and reproductive health.

The need to integrate HIV and RH policy, programming, and service delivery is accepted in principle. What does this consensus mean in real terms for donors and governments, service users, and providers?

## Synergies between HIV/AIDS and Reproductive Health Programs and Services

Closer examination of the content of reproductive health and HIV/AIDS programs reveals not only many reasons for linking them, but also a host of opportunities to do so. Lule (2004) points out that both types of programs "address human sexuality, serve similar target groups, promote safe and responsible sexual behavior, treat sexually transmitted infections, rely on prevention, and promote and distribute condoms within and outside clinics and health services."

Table 5.1 highlights the typical components of family planning programs, maternal and child health programs, and HIV/STI programs. The comparison yields evident synergies between these types of programs. Reproductive health and HIV/AIDS programs both require and use similar medical/health skills and facilities and rely on community participation to address sensitive sexuality issues and sociocultural determinants of behavior change. Both have shared objectives and desire the same outcomes, including reductions in maternal, infant, and child mortality. Both are interested in addressing the vulnerability and high-risk behaviors of young people that fuel the HIV epidemic in their age group and contribute to early childbearing and high maternal and infant mortality. Moreover, both focus and rely on behavior change and employ similar behavior change communication channels.

There are also challenges and limitations to achieving effective synergies between the two program areas. First, and most important, many groups

**Table 5.1**  *Typical Components of Family Planning, Maternal and Child Health, and HIV/STI Programs*

*Family planning/pregnancy prevention*

- Counseling and IEC
- Provision of contraceptives and condom distribution
- Basic screening of STIs and reproductive tract infections
- Infection prevention and quality of care
- Youth-friendly services
- Male involvement
- Community participation

*Maternal and child health*

- Antenatal and newborn care
- Safe delivery
- Emergency obstetric care
- PMTCT
- Breastfeeding support
- Well baby and well child care
- Postabortion care
- Community participation

*HIV/STI*

- Behavior change through IEC, counseling, and reducing stigma and discrimination
- Condom promotion and distribution
- Voluntary counseling and testing
- Diagnosis and treatment of STIs
- Prevention of PMTCT
- Treatment with antivirals
- Male involvement and youth-targeted programs
- Treatment, care, and support
- Community participation
- Health worker safety
- Social safety net

*Source:* Author.
IEC = information, education, and communication; PMTCT = prevention of mother-to-child transmission.

that are at high risk of becoming infected (youth, men, sex workers, and increasingly the partners of men in vulnerable groups) do not use reproductive health services that are geared to serve mothers and children.

## Competition for Resources

Many of the countries hardest hit by HIV/AIDS already had weak health systems, the human and organizational resources of which were further undermined by the epidemic. These systems have not always been able to readily and effectively utilize the large influx of AIDS funding. Meanwhile, the competition for human and organizational resources between parallel programs may have undermined the systems' capacity to deliver reproductive health services.

Historically, family planning and maternal and child health programs have been organized vertically and have tended not to target people at risk of becoming infected with HIV for many reasons. First, before the epidemic became widespread among the general population, those most at risk belonged on the whole to groups not traditionally served by family planning and maternal and child health services, such as men (including men who have sex with men), drug users, and commercial sex workers. Second, because of the stigma associated with the disease it was felt that offering HIV/AIDS services in the same place as family planning and maternal and child health services might dissuade those seeking antenatal care and other reproductive health services. However, those providing HIV/AIDS services feel that they have had to work hard to achieve recognition of the seriousness of the epidemic and for funding to fight it; some are reluctant to work with programs that they consider latecomers to the effort.

In the late 1990s there was increasing competition between HIV/AIDS and reproductive health programs for donor financial support. In the period 1995–2001, despite the increasing world population, funding for family planning dipped, while support for other reproductive health services remained static; and both declined in real terms. Meanwhile, support for HIV, and STIs generally, rose eightfold (Gillespie 2003) (see figure 5.1).

This competition arose not simply because of HIV/AIDS but because of the huge increase in a range of health sector initiatives, including, for example, the Global Fund Against AIDS, Tuberculosis, and Malaria; the Global Alliance for Vaccines and Immunization; the Global Alliance for Improved Nutrition; the International AIDS Vaccine, International Trachoma, and Global Polio Eradication initiatives; the Rollback Malaria and Stop TB partnerships; and the Guinea Worm Eradication and Lymphatic Filariasis Elimination programs.

**Figure 5.1** *Population Assistance from All Donors, 1995–2001*

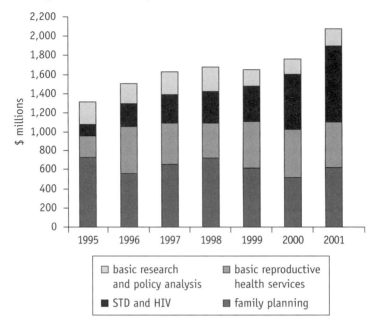

*Source:* Gillespie 2003.

Since 2001 the funding for reproductive health has further declined. Figure 5.2 shows how foundation funding (excluding funding for HIV/AIDS) in developing countries decreased significantly in 2002.

Projections of donor funding of reproductive health commodities (figure 5.3) show a growing deficit that could threaten achievement of some MDGs (Population Action International 2001).

## Commonality of Entry Points

The commonality of entry points for both HIV and reproductive health must surely outweigh these negative signs. Eight joint entry points are offered here: behavior change for safer sex, male involvement, community awareness, adolescent health, dual protection, family planning needs of HIV-positive women, prevention of mother-to-child transmission (PMTCT), and voluntary and confidential counseling and treatment (VCCT).

**Figure 5.2** *Foundations' Funding for Reproductive Health (Excluding HIV/AIDS) in Developing Countries, 1999–2002*

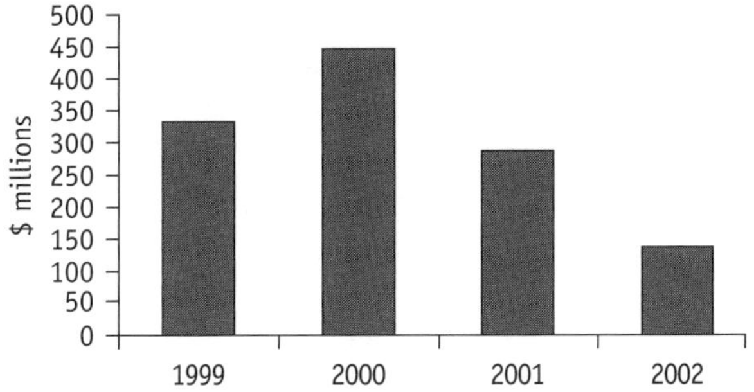

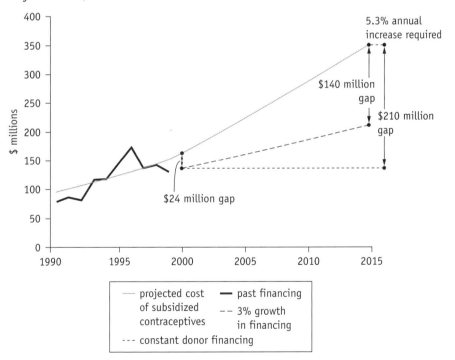

*Source:* Funders Network on Population, Reproductive Health and Rights. http://www.fundersnet.org (accessed 16 October 2003).

**Figure 5.3** *Donor Financing for Reproductive Health Commodities versus Projected Need, 1990–2015*

*Source:* Population Action International 2001.

## Behavior Change for Safer Sex

Achieving behavior change means dealing with the highly sensitive topic of sexuality that leads to risk and vulnerability. This effort involves exploring the nature of sexual behavior and underlying motives—from both partners' perspective and in premarital, marital, and extramarital situations. The motives—pressure (individual, group, or societal), pleasure, pain, and procreation—are difficult to research, discuss, and influence. Moreover, work on behavior change has to address the attitudes and needs of both women and men.

Family planning and maternal and child health clinicians have not traditionally been trained to tackle the taboo subjects of sexuality and sexual preference, as well as other sensitive topics associated with sexual behavior. Front-line workers at VCCT clinics are well placed to do so because family planning, maternal and child health, and VCCT services are often the same, particularly in countries that have a generalized effort. It is therefore sensible and efficient—even cost-effective—to offer integrated services performed by health workers with the necessary skills to deal with clients requiring both types of services, while recognizing that time may need to be set aside for the provision of services to particular groups—men, adolescents, commercial sex workers—not otherwise disposed to make use of a "one-stop shop."

As discussed below, an understanding of the different ways in which men and women may view sexuality and reproduction is another important factor in education for behavior change.

## Male Involvement

Male involvement in behavior change is crucial, but not easy to attain. First, men neither menstruate nor bear children, nor do they usually play the major role in child rearing; hence, they are less accustomed than women to discussing medical issues associated with fertility, pregnancy, childbirth, and general health. Second, both sexes are to a large extent constrained by the sociocultural context in which they have been raised. Generally speaking, girls are brought up with expectations to be feminine, nonaggressive, innocent, submissive, ready to please men, and bear children, for whom they are expected to care, whereas boys are expected to be risk takers and sexually assertive and to nurture the "weaker sex." Women who carry condoms are viewed as promiscuous rather than as well prepared; men are expected to know everything about sex and not need to ask. Men are expected to be macho and have multiple partners; women are expected to be pure and good mothers. This socialization of the sexes and resulting gender roles make both sexes vulnerable to HIV/AIDS infection and put women at risk of unwanted pregnancy and STIs.

Given the social pressure to conform to these stereotypes, it is hardly surprising that persuading men to ask for help in protecting themselves and their partners is difficult. Men are more accustomed to boast about their sexual conquests than to discuss the intimate details of their sexual life that relate to the use of condoms for family planning or assessment of their risk when it comes to HIV/AIDS. Finding ways to involve men in the design and delivery of services aimed at both sexes and in the provision of special services that target male needs is crucial.

## Community Awareness

Chapter 6 examines the case of a woman, Safar Banu, who died following childbirth, in an analysis of the importance of the role played by the community when it comes to influencing actions in the health sector. In that case, the community was actively involved in deciding if Safar should be taken to hospital and thus to some extent bears part of the responsibility for the health outcome that ensued. In nearly every country, communities have been mobilized to fight the AIDS pandemic. The challenge therefore is to ensure that communities understand the nature of the relationship between HIV/AIDS and reproductive health and that messages are integrated where possible and, when not, that they are mutually reinforcing.

## Adolescent Health

The fastest growing HIV epidemic is among 15-to-24-year olds; 50 percent of all new infections occur among this age group. In addition, early sexual activity exposes adolescents to unwanted pregnancy and higher degrees of attendant complications. For decades reproductive health practitioners have been working to get the appropriate information and services to this hard-to-reach group. Advocates of integrated HIV/AIDS and reproductive health programs should build on successful efforts to target the group (in Uganda and Sri Lanka, for example) and tailor their activities to provide joint messages and services.

## Dual Protection

Where services are separated, STI clients tend to be offered condoms for STI/HIV prevention, whereas family planning clients are offered barrier methods, including the condom, for birth spacing. If, for whatever reason, services have to remain separated, the message of dual protection against both pregnancy and STIs should still be conveyed. This message is especially important in countries where the HIV epidemic is becoming more generalized. For example, in Cambodia 42 percent of all new HIV infections occur via transmission from husbands to wives, while about one-third of new infections occur in babies born to these women (Hall and Chhoung 2005). In this situation, there is an urgent need to persuade women who may be at risk of infection from their husbands' extramarital activities to use the condom, ostensibly for birth spacing but also as a means of preventing STIs.

## Family Planning Needs of HIV-Positive Women

Women with immune-compromised systems are at higher risk than healthy women of complications arising from pregnancy and delivery—to say nothing of the potential risks to the infant of contracting HIV from its mother in utero, through childbirth, or through breastfeeding. By planning pregnancy, HIV-positive women can minimize the risk of infection for both their partner and child. For example, they can ensure that intercourse occurs when their CD4 count (a measure of their immune system) is high and viral load is low (indicating a low level of infection and therefore the least risk of infection for the man) and when they have access to antiretrovirals in the last few months of pregnancy and their infants can be given them at birth. Clearly, an HIV-positive woman wishing to become pregnant needs to be able to avail herself of the most accurate and up-to-date information regarding her options.

Contraceptive choice is also needed to avoid abortion. Where modern contraceptive methods are readily available, abortion rates fall, as illustrated in figure 5.4, which shows the total abortion rate and the prevalence of modern contraceptive methods in 18 countries (Westoff 2003).

As table 5.2 shows, both HIV-positive women and HIV-negative women are less likely to become pregnant if they are offered, and use, a modern method of contraception.

Strong arguments can be made for the provision of family planning services within the context of HIV/AIDS services aimed at women who seek screening for HIV or who are already HIV-positive and seek treatment, care, or both.

**Figure 5.4** Total Abortion Rate and the Prevalence of Modern Contraceptive Methods in 18 Countries

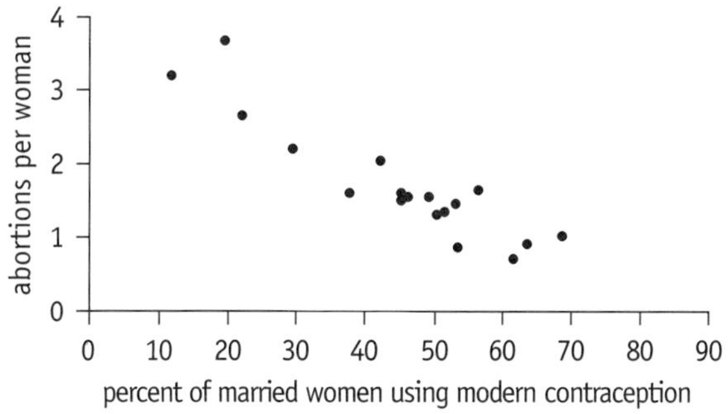

Source: Westoff 2003.

**Table 5.2** Incidence of Pregnancy Before and After a Family Planning Intervention

|  | Before (1988–90) | After (1992–93) |
|---|---|---|
| HIV-positive women | 22 percent (n = 402) | 9 percent (n = 311) |
| HIV-negative women | 30 percent (n = 934) | 20 percent (n = 159) |

Source: King and others 1995.

## Prevention of Mother-to-Child Transmission

PMTCT is a common entry point. The Mother and Child HIV Initiative currently covers 14 countries. Table 5.3 summarizes the expected costs and benefits of PMTCT and family planning services in 2007 in those countries as expressed in terms of child HIV infections and child deaths averted, number of orphans averted, mothers' lives saved, and costs of treatment.

With or without HIV, the risk to mother and baby is high when birth intervals are low (Rutstein 2000). Therefore advice on birth spacing is of importance not just to HIV-negative women but even more so to women with weakened immune systems due to HIV infection and AIDS-related opportunistic infections.

## Voluntary and Confidential Counseling and Treatment

Most countries now offer some form of VCCT services, usually through specialized clinics that deliver pretest and posttest counseling combined with services aimed at helping those with a negative test result to maintain their

**Table 5.3** Expected Costs and Benefits of PMTCT in the 14 Countries Covered by the Mother and Child HIV Initiative in 2007

| | Child HIV infections averted | Child deaths averted | Orphans averted | Mothers' lives saved |
|---|---|---|---|---|
| PMTCT | 38,000 | 19,000 | | |
| | 10,000–70,000 | 6,000–34,000 | | |
| PMTCT cost per event averted | $1,300 | $2,500 | | |
| | $350–$2,200 | $700–$4,400 | | |
| Family planning at PMTCT and VCCT sites | 48,000 | 97,000 | 232,000 | 16,000 |
| | 20,000–70,000 | 60,000–130,000 | 130,000–330,000 | 10,000–22,000 |
| Family planning cost per event averted | $990 | $450 | $200 | $2,800 |
| | $180–$1,800 | $200–$710 | $60–$330 | $1,300–$4,300 |

*Source:* Stover 2003.

negative status. The latter services include advice on condom use and provision of condoms. For those with a positive test result, appropriate referrals are made as necessary. Because family planning services are unlikely to be able to offer STI detection and testing, clients are referred to STI clinics. There is a strong argument for the provision of HIV testing where blood is routinely taken (for example, ANCs) and for clients at VCCT clinics to receive advice on birth spacing, together with products, when required.

## Sexually Transmitted Infections

Although HIV is not exclusively transmitted through sexual activity,[9] it is one of many sexually transmitted infections. In 2000, there were an estimated 340 million new cases among adults of curable STIs (including gonorrhea, chlamydia, syphilis, and trichomoniasis). As table 5.4 shows, the highest concentration of these STIs is in South and Southeast Asia.

In the past, services for these infections have been directed toward men and have been more in the form of treatment rather than prevention. All too often men have resorted to dermatologists, private sector providers, and over-the-counter medicines. However, HIV/AIDs research in the 1980s revealed high levels of STIs among women, a close link between STIs and HIV (partly as cofactors and partly because a person with an STI is more vulnerable to HIV infection), and the importance of STI control as an HIV prevention strategy.

**Table 5.4** *Worldwide Distribution of Curable STIs*

| Region | Millions |
| --- | :---: |
| Australasia | 1 |
| East Asia and Pacific | 18 |
| Eastern Europe and Central Asia | 22 |
| Latin America and the Caribbean | 38 |
| North Africa and Middle East | 10 |
| North America | 14 |
| South and Southeast Asia | 151 |
| Sub-Saharan Africa | 69 |
| Western Europe | 17 |
| **Total** | **340** |

*Source:* WHO 2001.

These findings led to intense efforts to integrate syndromic management into antenatal care and family planning services in the 1990s, but low effectiveness discouraged further efforts. This low effectiveness was in part due to increasing attention to HIV/AIDS at the expense of STI management and other reproductive health services, and in part because integrated services did not easily reach adolescents, unmarried persons, men in general, and sex workers.

Even so, scope for reproductive health services to include HIV and STIs remains. For example, antenatal, family planning, and child health services are relatively accessible and increasingly utilized. Clients of these services may be receptive to HIV information, which they can pass on, and to services, to which they can refer others. Antenatal clinics and delivery and postpartum services also provide opportunities to prevent perinatal and breastfeeding HIV transmission. And, in a more generalized HIV epidemic, where, because of her partner's behavior, a married woman may no longer be "low risk," she will have ready access to advice and services that could help her prevent HIV infection.

## Collaboration and Integration

Key HIV/AIDS services that can be provided through reproductive health services include education on safer sex (including education on HIV and STIs), referrals for voluntary confidential counseling and testing, encouragement of condom use for double protection and supply of condoms, PMTCT, counseling and testing of pregnant women for HIV and other conditions, supply of antiretrovirals, prevention and treatment of STIs, and care for people living with HIV/AIDS. Such services would help ensure that persons testing HIV-positive have access to a full range of contraceptive services, including sterilization and, where legal, safe abortion, while persons testing negative would be fully supported to maintain their status by promoting dual protection. Figure 5.5 illustrates the potential integration of HIV/AIDS and reproductive health services for a variety of individuals.

⟨The programmatic strengths of reproductive health are principally the long experience of service providers in program design and management. These providers know how to maximize the use of key stakeholders, including religious leaders, youth, parliamentarians, and politicians, to advocate for reproductive health. But reproductive health champions have had little success at drawing sustained attention to reproductive health issues at the highest political levels. When the international development goals became the MDGs, the specific goal relating to reproductive health was dropped. AIDS activists, on the other hand, have succeeded in helping set the AIDS agenda at the highest level. Perhaps one of the ways in which they have managed to do this is by strategically focusing attention on the economic issues that go hand in glove with the HIV/AIDS pandemic. Reproductive health advocates are heeding this lesson as they increasingly use the burden

**Figure 5.5**  *Potential Integration of HIV/AIDS and Reproductive Health Services for a Variety of Individuals*

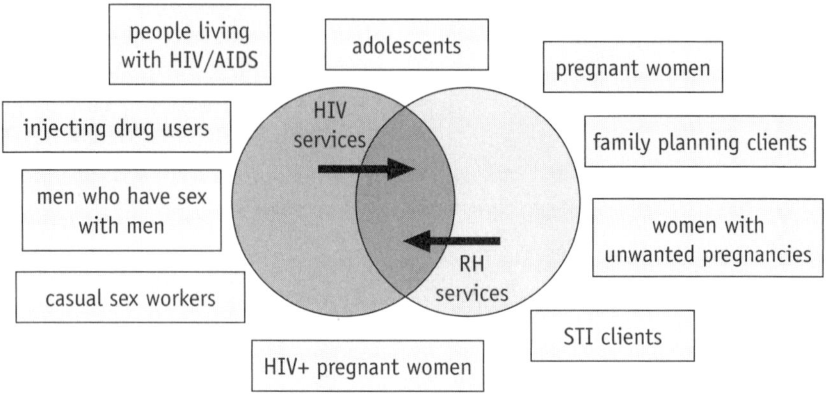

*Source:* Author.

of reproductive ill health, and its commensurate impact on household resources, to draw greater attention to the links between poverty and reproductive health status. Because community and religious leaders, parliamentarians, and so on have been so effective in championing the AIDS cause, reproductive health advocates should seize the opportunity to link their cause to that of HIV/AIDS and to advocate for integrated reproductive health and HIV/AIDS policies, programs, and services. The message should be that HIV/AIDS and reproductive health are symbiotic: where one is being addressed, so should the other.

## An Obstacle to Integration?

A possible obstacle to integration of reproductive health and HIV/AIDS initiatives is practical and political issues resulting from application of the "Mexico City" policy—also known as the "global gag rule"—to health sector assistance. Unlike other health funding, global AIDS funding appears to be exempt from the rule, but workers in the field may be unaware that this is the case because of the absence of clear guidance on the matter. Moreover, confusion is understandable because there is no programmatic, moral, or ethical rationale for waiving the gag rule for HIV/AIDS ("to save lives") but enforcing it for contraception, even at the cost of untold lives lost to pregnancy and related causes, including unsafe abortion—lives that could unquestionably be saved by facilitating access to family planning services impeded by imposition of the rule. Opposition to certain elements of the ICPD Program of Action by those with conservative attitudes toward family planning and abortion poses a risk to both vertical and integrated programs and creates yet one more hazard for service providers to navigate.

## Conclusion

A two-pronged approach would be most effective for improving maternal and child health and tackling HIV/AIDS. One prong is to promote reproductive health services as the main health services contact point for women and children and to increase the availability and improve the quality of those services so as to improve the acceptability, coverage, and efficiency of PMTCT programs and thus reduce the spread of HIV. The other prong is to promote the collaboration and, to the extent feasible, the integration of HIV/AIDS services and programs with reproductive health services and programs.

Combined efforts will stand a better chance of succeeding in a world where many health systems are weak; VCCT uptake is low; HIV/AIDS and other reproductive health ailments are a major burden; access to HIV care, support, and treatment is limited; community and male partner involvement is low or lacking; and stigma and discrimination persist.

Horizons must be expanded so that combined services reach core and bridging populations, including men, sex workers, and adolescents. For men, the aim must be to promote their use of condoms, encourage them to accompany their partners to health service centers, and reach men who have sex with men. For sex workers and adolescents, the aim must be to provide access to routine services and to improve providers' understanding of their needs. Meeting these goals means strengthening community-based services that will educate people about HIV, sexually transmitted diseases, and protection. Such services will promote the use of VCCT and will provide care for those living with HIV/AIDS.

# PART II

## Tools for Adapting to Change

# 6

## *Pressure Points: Using the Pathways Framework*

Every year more than half a million maternal deaths and around 4 million perinatal deaths occur in low- and middle-income countries, mostly among the poorest groups within these countries. An even larger toll of morbidities (more than 8 million each year) results from nonfatal complications of delivery. Most of these deaths and disabilities are preventable, and the interventions required to prevent them are known. The sad reality is that in many instances effective reproductive health interventions are either not available to poor women or so poor in quality that they are ineffective.

This chapter focuses on obstacles that prevent poor women from benefiting from the knowledge and technical expertise that is available and on the factors beyond care that shape reproductive health outcomes. It employs an adapted version of the "pathways" framework from the World Bank's guidelines for Poverty Reduction Strategy Papers to link factors at various levels—individuals, households, and communities and government policies in health and other sectors—that directly or indirectly affect reproductive health outcomes. Figure 6.1 depicts this simple framework for assessing the impact of factors inside and outside the health system that influence health, including reproductive health.

These factors operate at several levels: (1) households and communities; (2) the health system (including health care, health finance, and health promotion) and sectors other than health such as education, nutrition, infrastructure (water and sanitation, transport, and communications) that directly or indirectly influence health outcomes; and (3) public policies and

**Figure 6.1** *Pathways to Reproductive Health Outcomes*

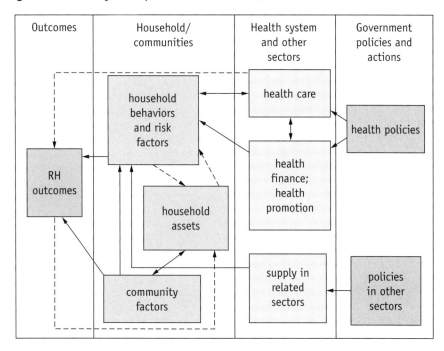

Source: Adapted from Claeson and others 2002.

actions that affect health systems and outcomes directly (health reforms, for example) or indirectly (macroeconomic policies).

## Households Behaviors and Resources

Good health is dependent not only on the provision of good medical services but also on healthy behavior and adequate household resources. Healthy behavior means avoiding or minimizing risks (for example, practicing family planning and safe sex). Such behavior requires knowledge about how to prevent disease and promote health as well as the ability to act on this information. Many health-promoting behaviors (for example, dietary habits, sanitary practices, fertility regulation, childcare, and utilization of health services) occur within families.

Household resources and assets (including income); the health and education of household members; access to water and sanitation, roads, and communication; and membership in formal and informal support networks also affect health outcomes. They influence behaviors and health risks—for example, whether or not to seek health care or act in response to health information. Economists view these household-level characteristics as demand-side, rather than supply-side, factors (Ensor and Cooper 2004).

Although it is common to treat all members of a family or household as a single unit, assuming that whatever benefits one member will benefit the entire household, it is widely acknowledged that intrahousehold differences in gender and age may significantly affect how decisions are made and whether a decision is beneficial for all members (Case and Deaton 2002). Thus, an understanding of household decision making is critical to an understanding of how policy decisions affect the welfare of families and individual family members.

Gender disparities in access to education, credit, and political influence have a considerable impact on how individual family members are valued and on the degree to which women as well as men have a voice in household decision making. Recognition of the importance of individuals and households in producing good (or poor) reproductive health outcomes should lead policy makers to focus on the constraints faced by vulnerable households and vulnerable members within those households.

## Community Factors

Household-level behaviors and risk factors are influenced and reinforced by conditions in the community. Community factors include both the values and norms that shape household attitudes and behaviors and the physical and environmental conditions of the community—for example, terrain and weather conditions that affect households' capacity to produce better outcomes.

Community factors that typically influence health outcomes are

- gender norms (which are influenced by social and cultural values) that shape the roles of and relationships between men and women;
- community groups that effectively (a) provide social cohesion (sometimes called social capital), which in turn supports positive behaviors in individuals and families, and (b) organize actions to improve health outcomes directly (community health insurance or pooling of resources to transport emergency cases) or indirectly (microcredit programs);
- community access to public services (inside and outside the health sector); and
- environmental conditions (safe water and location—distance from a health facility, terrain, weather conditions).

Gender deserves special attention because of the inequity in social relationships that restricts the rights of women to make decisions for themselves or to have fair access to household assets. The greater the inequity, the greater the obstacle to poor women's access to lifesaving interventions.

## Health System Obstacles

Improvement of reproductive health outcomes requires a continuum of care, from the household and community through the referral process to an effectively functioning health system. In addition to health care, other health system factors—finance, information, and management of input— can influence health outcomes.

Cost may create a financial obstacle to poor women's access to care. Costs include direct payments for care and transport as well as opportunity cost—for example, lost wages or time that otherwise would have been spent in household production. Even when publicly provided care is nominally free, under-the-table or side payments may be required to obtain services or medicines. Evidence suggests that the poor already pay a lot out of pocket, particularly for medicines, and could obtain better care for their money if health system performance were improved (Nahar and Costello 1998). Financial obstacles can be reduced through subsidies, insurance schemes, and exemptions that effectively target the poor.

Health education, including behavior change communication, can play an important role in informing individuals and households about health risks and how to avoid them, letting them know about available health interventions and their benefits, and instructing them in practices such as hand washing and utilization of oral rehydration.

Effective management of health system inputs, including availability of medicines, training and deployment of health workers, and the location and maintenance of health facilities, also affect health outcomes.

Poor health system performance is one of the reasons that poor women do not benefit from lifesaving reproductive health interventions—for example, when they experience an obstetric complication. A cross-national review of health system failures that contributed to high maternal mortality identified several critical problems: shortage of trained personnel, lack of equipment and facilities (including consumables such as blood products and antibiotics), and poor patient management (Sundari 1992). These problems were also pinpointed in the World Bank's assessment of obstacles to the achievement of health-related Millennium Development Goals (MDGs). The report mentions the quality of care as reflected in health workforce performance, availability of medicines, and inadequate and ineffective public spending. A review of the benefit incidence of public spending on health care in Africa found that subsidies are poorly targeted and typically favor the better off, a phenomenon not limited to Africa (Castro-Leal and others 1999).

## Related Sectors

Other sectors that affect reproductive health outcomes include transportation, education, and water and sanitation.

### Transportation

For women who experience an obstetric emergency, delays in reaching a treatment facility can be life threatening. Such delays can be the result of physical accessibility factors such as distance to a facility, the availability and cost of transport, and the condition of roads, all of which affect the time required to get a mother to a facility once the decision to seek care has been made (Thaddeus and Maine 1994).

### Education

Education of women influences reproductive health in a variety of ways, including attitudes toward childbearing, health-seeking behaviors, and earning opportunities. Early gains in female literacy played an important role in maternal mortality ratio (MMR) declines in Malaysia and Sri Lanka (Pathmanathan 2003). A review of the impact of education on autonomy and reproductive behavior revealed that education enhances women's knowledge about the outside world and increases their awareness of the importance of family health and hygiene and of the treatment and prevention of illness (Jejeebhoy 1995). Another consequence noted by the review was greater decision-making autonomy within the home. However, contextual factors can influence the impact of education on women's participation in household decision making; a society characterized by a high degree of gender stratification is likely to weaken that participation (Jejeebhoy 1995).

### Water and Sanitation

Provision of safe water has been cited as a factor in declines of mortality in developed countries (van Poppel and van der Heijden 1997). Lack of sanitation and safe water, along with poor personal hygiene, are known to be major factors in the wide prevalence of parasitic diseases in poor countries. Studies of the impact of safe water on infant and childhood mortality typically do not focus separately on neonatal mortality, but they recognize that waterborne diseases can undermine the health of pregnant women because they cause anemia, a risk factor for mothers as well as their newborns. One report cites unsafe water supply as well as pollutants from fuels used in cooking as risk factors in the high MMRs of the African countries studied (Santiso 1997; Paul 1993). There is a sharp difference in the percent of households with safe water in the countries with MMRs under 30 (92 percent) compared with those with MMRs over 1,000 (51 percent). The link between water supply and MMRs/neonatal mortality ratios involves both household and community factors. A household's consumption of water may be constrained by prices, income, and other household variables even if water is supplied at the community level. Jalan and Ravallion (2001) have observed that health gains largely bypassed poor children when piped water was available in their community, particularly when the mother was poorly educated.

## Nutrition

Poor nutrition is another key factor in maternal and neonatal mortality. Poor nutrition and closely spaced births are closely linked to maternal and neonatal mortality. In India anemia is reported to be an indirect factor in 64.4 percent of maternal deaths (Buckshee 1997). As the Safar Banu case (box 6.1) demonstrates, gender stratification and attitudes can also contribute to poor nutrition by depriving poor women of adequate nutrition not only during pregnancy but also during childhood and adolescence, leading to small stature and a higher risk of delivery complications.

## Government Policies and Actions

Government policies and actions can affect both the health system and other sectors that influence reproductive health outcomes. Most countries are implementing reforms to improve health system performance. Reforms include changes in organization and accountability, revenue generation, and allocation and purchasing, as well as regulation. Policies and actions in other sectors also affect health because of their influence on attitudes and behavior and on the supply of related services such as education, transport, water, and food security. Taxation can also influence health behaviors—for example, "sin taxes" on tobacco and alcohol discourage use of those substances.

Health reformers have argued that cost recovery could improve the sustainability, quality, and equity of health services by bringing payments into the open, rationalizing consumption of services (for example, through incentives to use the level of care appropriate for the treatment required), and giving providers control over resources and the incentive to employ resources to improve quality. Cost recovery, combined with effective exemption schemes for the poor, could redirect public subsidies that typically benefit the rich more than the poor.

Evaluating the impact of cost recovery schemes on maternal and neonatal health outcomes for the poor is not an easy task because of the many contextual and institutional influences that shape their implementation. In a review of experience with user fees in Africa, where many countries introduced them during the 1980s, Gilson (1997) reported the following:

- By themselves, fees tend to dissuade the poor more than the rich from using services.
- Fees, especially for community-managed schemes such as the Bamako Initiative that focus on medicines, may be associated with quality improvements that offset some of that negative impact on utilization.
- The equity impact depends a lot on the nature of the payment mechanism—direct payments have a more negative effect.
- Fees do not appear to generate sufficient revenue to enable the hoped-for reallocation of public subsidies to the poor.
- Exemption schemes do not really protect the poor and often help other groups (for example, public sector employees) more than the poor.
- Differential geographic implementation of fee schedules may only exacerbate geographic inequalities in access to care.
- Evidence of fees' impact on poor households' budgets and demand for health care is very limited.

Research shows that poor households' service use substantially drops immediately after fees' introduction and later increases, but not to pre fee levels. Poor households are somewhat more sensitive to price changes than better-off households.

Other macroeconomic policies can affect reproductive health outcomes. For example, tariffs, taxes, and price controls on health system inputs (medicines, equipment, water, and electricity) can limit the access of poor people. Budget and personnel ceilings required by macroeconomic stabilization programs may limit the capacity of the health sector to provide services, even when financing is available. And policies affecting employment or agricultural production may limit poor households' capacity to access health care.

**Box 6.1** *Why Did Safar Banu Die?*

Safar Banu, age 43, never attended an antenatal clinic. She said she had already given birth to nine children without the help of a clinic. Why should she need antenatal checkups now? She was too busy and had no time for such visits. While several months pregnant, she worked in the fields shredding jute fibers, work usually performed only by the poorest women. Safar Banu did not use contraceptives. She wished to use them, but her husband threatened to divorce her if she did. According to her mother, Safar cried when she became pregnant for the 10th time. The pregnancy itself did not present special problems, but during the last month Safar complained of swollen feet and dizziness. A week before giving birth, she felt very weak and told her mother she feared she would not survive the birth. At the time, her anemic condition, which later became obvious, was not recognized by her family.

Safar Banu's husband held a great deal of faith in Gopal Daktar (the local healer). Daktar was called at the onset of labor and gave two tablets to increase labor contractions. After the birth, he again gave medicine to reduce the pain. All of these tablets were just aspirin, which Daktar admitted when later interviewed. At the delivery, Safar's mother was present with the *dai* (traditional birth attendant). The birth was difficult because Safar was so weak. After the birth, she was unable to get up for 10 hours. The *dai* and her mother knew that something was seriously wrong. The husband did not realize that his wife's condition had deteriorated. He became alarmed only on the fifth day, when Safar's entire body became swollen.

The women in the village explained Safar's headaches by the blood that had risen from her womb to her head. They view this blood as polluted and therefore as extremely harmful if it goes to the head.

It appears that Safar lost a considerable amount of blood after giving birth. The loss did not cause much concern, because she was considered not to have bled long enough. Thus, she did not completely eliminate the polluted blood that was believed to be the cause of her swelling.

On the fifth day, Safar had a sensation of burning in her limbs and asked for water to be poured over her head for the entire day. She was sweating profusely

## Case Study: Why Did Safar Banu Die?

The case study in box 6.1 illustrates the obstacles that typically prevent poor women from obtaining lifesaving interventions when they suffer an obstetric complication. The case is taken from an oral autopsy conducted in Bangladesh during the early 1990s that played an important role in shaping the development of a maternal health strategy for Bangladesh later in

**Box 6.1** *Why Did Safar Banu Die? (continued)*

but registered no fever. Two days before she died, a midwife from the maternal and child health clinic was called. She recommended that Safar be transferred immediately to the district hospital. She diagnosed a case of extreme anemia and thought that a blood transfusion was necessary and urgent. The husband did not listen to the midwife. He had more confidence in Gopal Daktar, who tried various medications and injections but to no avail. Daktar later claimed that he gave no "good" (meaning expensive) medicines because the family was too poor to pay. Daktar was annoyed with the family for wasting his time.

On the seventh day, Safar Banu became unconscious. Her mother had her carried to the maternal and child health clinic to get treatment from the midwife. Safar's condition had deteriorated considerably, and it was feared that she would not survive the night. Her pulse was extremely low, and she had difficulty breathing. The clinic offered to pay for medicines, but transport to hospital was to be the family's responsibility, according to the official policy. At this point, the elder son and a cousin took charge of the affair. They organized and paid for transport to the district hospital. Safar's mother felt that it was probably too late and attempted to discourage her grandson. Half a *kani* of land had to be sold to pay for transport, and the husband is still bitter with the clinic for not having provided any financial help. The son gave his own blood to save his mother but to no avail. The husband, a sick man himself, never went to the hospital. Safar Banu died the following day.

Safar Banu's mother confirmed how late the husband became aware of his wife's critical state. Mention was also made of how hard Safar worked and how little she ate after her husband and sons had been fed. She drank water when there was no rice. When she was ill in the past, she had returned to her mother, a poor woman herself, to get help and treatment. The husband only thought of his own illness and did not see his wife's problems. Safar Banu knew how to bear her sorrows in silence. Her husband praised her because she was uncomplaining.

*Source:* Blanchet 1991.

that decade. It describes the plight of a poor woman, Safar Banu, who died as a result of complications during her 10th delivery. Although the midwife diagnosed Safar's condition as "extreme anemia," and the symptoms also suggest septicemia (once a leading cause of maternal deaths and now rare in richer countries), the case reveals a complex of causes of Safar Banu's death.

A complex interplay of forces (typical of those that affect poor women around the world) undermined Safar Banu's chances of survival in the face of a life-threatening obstetric emergency. They included

- Safar's subordinate status in the household and willingness to endure this status;
- her nonuse of contraception and lack of voice in this decision;
- her poor nutritional status as the last and least fed in her household;
- her lack of antenatal care despite swelling and dizziness;
- her household's inability to pay for medicines;
- her husband's refusal to listen to the midwife and reliance on the advice of the traditional healer, who failed to provide adequate care;
- misinformation about Safar's condition, which delayed treatment at the clinic; and
- transport costs, for which the family had to sell land (creating a legacy of resentment) and which further delayed treatment.

A combination of circumstances, mostly outside the health system, was the cause of Safar's death. Those circumstances reflect many of the household- and community-level factors that contribute to maternal and neonatal mortality. The household factors are unequal gender relationships, behaviors relating to fertility regulation and nutrition, poor education and lack of information, and household poverty and inability to pay for care. The community factors are the gender culture, misinformation, and lack of community support.

But the potential of community mobilization to reduce maternal and neonatal mortality is also evident in the Safar Banu case. Many community mobilization initiatives are proving effective. They include involvement of community health workers in creating awareness about complications of delivery and demand for effective management of emergencies, community support for transport, and support for mothers during delivery.

# 7

## It Starts in the Household

The pathways framework, introduced by the World Bank (Claeson and others 2002) and described in chapter 6, has refocused attention on the critical role of the household in the production of good health. It might appear obvious that individual and family actions and decisions are instrumental in achieving health outcomes, but policy work and most resources in health sector budgets are typically targeted at the supply-side medical care elements of the health productions function. Very little attention is paid to the demand side of medical care.

### The Scientific Evidence

*The Millennium Development Goals for Health: Rising to the Challenges* (Wagstaff and Claeson 2004) summarized all available evidence on preventive and treatment interventions that are proven to be effective in reducing child and maternal mortality, lowering malnutrition, and addressing communicable diseases (HIV/AIDS, tuberculosis, and malaria). The list of effective interventions is reproduced in table 7.1.

Two of the main conclusions of *The Millennium Development Goals for Health* are that we already know what needs to be done to achieve the MDGs and that most of what needs to be done is low tech: "It is not the lack of interventions that is the main obstacle to faster progress toward the MDGs . . . Using all known interventions . . . could avert 63 percent of child deaths and 74 percent of maternal deaths" (Wagstaff and Claeson 2004).

**Table 7.1** *Effective Interventions for Reducing Illness, Death, and Malnutrition*

| Goal | Preventive interventions | Treatment interventions |
|---|---|---|
| Child mortality | Breastfeeding; hand washing; safe disposal of stool; latrine use; safe preparation of weaning foods; use of insecticide-treated nets; complementary feeding; immunization; micronutrient supplementation (zinc and vitamin A); antenatal care, including steroids and tetanus toxoid, antimalarial intermittent preventive treatment in pregnancy, newborn temperature management, nevirapine and replacement feeding, antibiotics for premature rupture of membranes, clean delivery. | Case management with oral rehydration therapy for diarrhea; antibiotics for dysentery, pneumonia, and sepsis; antimalarials for malaria; newborn resuscitation; breastfeeding; complementary feeding during illness; micronutrient supplementation (zinc and vitamin A). |
| Maternal mortality | Family planning (lifetime risk), intermittent malaria prophylaxis, use of insecticide-treated bed nets, micronutrient supplementation (iron, folic acid, calcium for those who are deficient). | Antibiotics for preterm rupture of membranes, skilled attendance (especially active management of third stage of labor), basic and emergency obstetric care. |
| Nutrition | Exclusive breastfeeding for 6 months, appropriate complementary child feeding for next 6–24 months, iron and folic acid supplementation for children, improved hygiene and sanitation, dietary intake of pregnant and lactating women, micronutrient supplementation for prevention of anemia and vitamin A deficiency for mothers and children, anthelminthic treatment in school-aged children. | Appropriate feeding of sick child and oral rehydration therapy, control and timely treatment of infectious and parasitic diseases, treatment and monitoring of severely malnourished children, high-dose treatment of clinical signs of vitamin A deficiency. |

*(continued)*

Another important conclusion of *The Millennium Development Goals for Health* is that households, in terms of actions and constraints, play the critical role in many if not most of these known interventions. Whether we are talking about breastfeeding, hand washing, preparation of meals, disposal of waste, use of bed nets, or sexual behavior, households play the key role. That is not to say that households are at fault if these preventive interventions do

**Table 7.1**  *(continued)*

| Goal | Preventive interventions | Treatment interventions |
|---|---|---|
| HIV/AIDS | Safe sex, including condom use; unused needles for drug users; treatment of sexually transmitted infections; safe, screened blood supplies. Antiretrovirals in pregnancy for PMTCT and after occupational exposure. | Treatment of opportunistic infections, cotrimoxazole prophylaxis, highly active antiretroviral therapy, palliative care. |
| Tuberculosis | Directly observed treatment of infectious cases to prevent transmission and emergence of drug-resistant strains and treatment of contacts, BCG (Calmette-Guérin bacillus) immunization. | Directly observed treatment to cure, including early identification of tuberculosis symptomatic cases. |
| Malaria | Use of insecticide-treated nets, indoor residual spraying (in epidemic-prone areas), intermittent presumptive treatment of pregnant women. | Rapid detection and early treatment of uncomplicated cases, treatment of complicated cases (such as cerebral malaria and severe anemia). |

*Source:* Wagstaff and Claeson 2004, table 3.1.

*Note:* "Intervention" means the direct action that leads to prevention or cure—a preventive measure, the management of a sick child, or a safe delivery. For example, the act of immunization rather than the vaccine is the intervention. Case management, not medicines or vitamins, is the intervention. Counseling for safer sex is not an intervention in this sense—safe sex is.

not occur. As we will see later in this chapter, and as was revealed in the Safar Banu case presented in chapter 6, many barriers stymie behavior change. Some of these barriers are financial in nature, others are cultural, and some relate to failures in the supply of critical inputs by health systems and other relevant sectors (chapter 13 addresses factors in sectors outside health).

## A Dual Role

One simple way to describe the role of individuals and households in table 7.1 is *consumer* of health services. With respect to maternal mortality interventions, for example, women can get access to attendants at deliveries or to emergency obstetric care. A more complete way of describing the role of individuals and households, however, is *producer* of overall health and well-being. In other words, households can be viewed as the units that combine inputs, such as preventive and curative health care as well as nutrition; that reduce risks through practices and decisions; and that ultimately produce good health.

If we accept households as producers of health, we need to empower them to be better producers of health. The first step is to understand the reasons that households often fail to behave in ways that are conducive to health. Constraints are unlikely to be universal and would need to be understood within the economic and cultural context of different countries and different parts of countries. Next, policies and resources should be aimed at eliminating constraints and facilitating more effective production of health, including better consumption of health services.

The international health community increasingly recognizes the importance of household actions and constraints, especially as they relate to access and use of health services. Box 7.1 gives examples of research findings in this area.

## Applying the Pathways Framework to the Safar Banu Case

Chapter 6 introduced the pathways framework and presented a case study of Safar Banu, a Bangladeshi woman who died during childbirth. Using the pathways framework, table 7.2 identifies the household and community factors that may have contributed to Safar Banu's death. As the table reveals, some factors are cross-cutting.

## Policy Implications

As noted above, many household and community factors influence reproductive health outcomes. Recognition of the influence of households and communities should be complemented by understanding of factors retarding households' production of good health. Once determinants of reproductive health outcomes are assessed, the policy question becomes what can be done to remove constraints (including negative cultural influences) to, and change behaviors for, households' production of good health.

The answer to this difficult policy question depends on many factors, such as the nature of the reproductive health problem in a given country, the country's capacity to influence household behavior or culture, and the availability

---

**Box 7.1** *Many Barriers to Improved Maternal Health and Survival are Behavioral*

- A study in Tanzania found that 21 percent of women delivered at home because of the rudeness of health staff—even though they thought delivering in a health facility was safer.
- Among the Saraguaro Indians in Ecuador (and many other traditional cultures), women perceive hospital-based deliveries as entailing a violation of privacy, unacceptable attendance by male providers, and unfamiliar birth positions.
- In Sudan a study found that many women were ashamed of being poorly dressed in front of health workers (who are generally of a higher socioeconomic class) and were afraid the health workers would react negatively to their illiteracy.
- In Ghana a study found that 64 percent of women who died of pregnancy-related complications had sought help from an herbalist, soothsayer, or other traditional provider before going to a health facility.
- In Nepal mothers-in-law attend most deliveries, and additional care or help is sought only if the mother-in-law decides that such care is needed.
- In Benin the government put significant pressure (including fines) on women to have institutional deliveries. But many women continued to deliver at home because of the honor brought to families if they were seen as "stoic" during labor and childbirth.

*Source:* Family Care International and the Safe Motherhood Inter-Agency Group 1998.

---

**Table 7.2** *Contributors to Safar Banu's Death*

| Household behaviors and risk factors | Household resources | Community factors |
|---|---|---|
| Decision not to use contraception | Limited financial resources delayed health-seeking behavior and transport | Religion reflected in household decision on contraception |
| Decision not to seek care from a qualified provider | Limited knowledge affected appropriate actions | Gender relations and the lack of women's voice within the household |
| Decisions about priority feeding when food is limited | Limited women's empowerment | Acceptance of traditional healers |
| Decision not to seek antenatal care | | |

*Source:* Authors.

of effective social mechanisms for mobilizing sustainable solutions. Increasingly, countries are experimenting with policies to address demand-side determinants. A few examples of apparently effective demand-side policies are highlighted below. Just because a policy works in one country, however, is no guarantee that it will work in another country.

### Expanding Outreach

As noted above, an important demand-side constraint to the use of lifesaving interventions is the inability to get access to services. A possible solution—and one that can address knowledge gaps as well—is expanding outreach. Outreach can take different forms, as evidenced by the vitamin A distribution strategies of three countries.

- *Nepal*—Implementation of its twice-yearly distribution for 6–59-month-olds was delegated to a nongovernmental organization. An existing cadre of female community health volunteers carries out the distribution.
- *Zambia*—Its distribution began with the National Immunization Day campaign. A decrease in national immunization days and rise in decentralization led to an extended outreach model and child health weeks. Vitamin A and other preventive services are provided through clinics, schools, and outreach sites designated by districts.
- *Ghana*—Its program began with National Integrated Development Strategies but led to mandated district experimentation. Neither schools alone nor clinic contacts proved sufficient as distribution networks. Now districts use a mix of clinics, schools, and house-to-house visits. They employ community mobilization and local progress assessments to adjust distribution strategies.

### Social Marketing

Another important factor in increasing the use of lifesaving services is to raise demand for these services. Many countries use social marketing to achieve this objective. Social marketing utilizes commercial marketing techniques and a progressive pricing approach to increase both demand for and physical access to effective services.

Social marketing of bed nets in Tanzania involved

- research into consumer preferences;
- creating product packaging that is attractive to the target client;
- setting a price that includes a subsidy;
- distributing discount vouchers for pregnant women and children;
- establishing sale points in every village in the targeted area; and
- implementing an aggressive promotion strategy that included posters, mobile videos, maternal and child health clinics, T-shirts, theater groups, and sports sponsorships.

### Conditional Cash Transfers

One of the most often cited reasons for lack of demand for important services is the inability to pay for them. A relatively new approach to increase demand for critical services by poor families is the use of conditional cash transfers. The idea is to pay poor families to send their kids to school and to demand and receive preventive health services. This approach was tested in Mexico.

- *Integrated health, education, and cash transfers to low-income families:*
    Universal cash transfer to all families (average $25/month)
    Education grant for families for grades P3 through S3
    Micronutrient-fortified foods for pregnant women and children
    Mandatory health services for pregnant women and children
- *Three-stage targeting:*
    Geographic—poor regions and communities
    Households—based on socioeconomic questionnaire
    Validation of selected households through public assembly
- *Coverage:*
    1997—initiation
    2000—2.6 million families (40 percent of all rural families)
    2004—4.5 million families (20 percent of total Mexican families)

## Conclusion

Outreach, social marketing, and conditional cash transfers are but three ways to address the role of households, eliminate barriers, and address cultural factors. Other possibilities include community-based planning and service delivery (for example, community-based planning for reproductive health services in Nepal [Malhotra and others 2005]), partnering with the private sector (for example, promotion of hand washing [see http://www.globalhandwashing.org/Publications/Attachments/WSP_H_Lessons_07Oct02.pdf]), and contracting for nongovernmental organizations (for example, contracting for primary care in Cambodia [Schwartz and Bhushan 2005]).

Simply working on service delivery from a system or supply-side perspective and ignoring factors that affect household actions, decisions, and constraints is unlikely to achieve the overall objective of improving health services.

# 8

## *Gender, Health, and Poverty*

Gender balance has a major bearing on health and poverty. Despite wider recognition of this fact, gender balance remains a sensitive subject in many parts of the world. Men make up half the population, and many of them prefer to avoid the topic, if only because they fear it may threaten their status. Women have a keener interest in the topic, because in many societies they continue to be subjugated by custom and culture.

Despite considerable progress in recent decades, gender inequalities remain pervasive in many dimensions of life. The most evident is in leadership. In only three countries (Andorra, Sweden, and the United States) did women hold at least 30 percent of government posts in 1996; 124 countries had governments that comprised fewer than 10 percent women, and 15 of those included no women at all. At that time the number of female ministers at cabinet level worldwide was 6.8 percent; in 48 countries, there were no female ministers.[10] Five years on, the position had hardly changed, as shown in the comparison in figure 8.1.

The cultural submission of women runs deep: every major religion in the world is male dominated. Although not addressed here, the impact of the lack of women in governance on the roles of men and women in the market and household economies that, in turn, influence health and poverty must be recognized.

Although disparities exist throughout the world, they tend to be more prevalent in poor developing countries. The differences in outcomes between men and women—and between boys and girls—are a consequence

**Figure 8.1** *Gender Disparity in Parliamentary Membership*

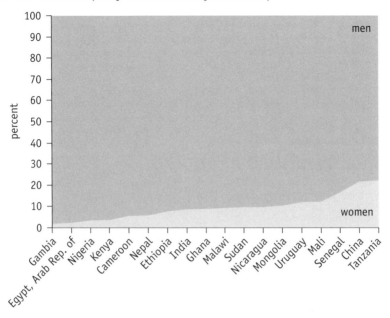

*Source:* Inter-Parliamentary Union 2001.

of differences in the opportunities and resources made available to them. Inequalities in the allocation of resources (such as education, health care, and nutrition) matter because of the strong association of these resources with well-being, productivity, and growth. The pattern of inequality begins at an early age, with boys routinely receiving a larger share of education and health spending than girls do. The female disadvantage is best reflected in differences in child mortality rates. Child mortality captures the effect of preferences for boys because adequate nutrition and medical interventions are particularly important for the one- to five-year age group. Given the natural female biological advantage, a female child mortality rate as high as or higher than a male child mortality rate suggests that girls are discriminated against.

The extent to which women and girls benefit from development policies and programs has a major impact on countries' overall development success. Research shows that women and girls tend to work harder than men, are more likely to invest their earnings in their children, are major producers as well as consumers, and shoulder life-sustaining responsibilities without which men and boys could not survive, much less enjoy high levels of productivity. Women's empowerment is particularly important for determining a country's demographic trends—trends that in turn affect a country's economic success and environmental sustainability.

Both men and women play substantial economic roles. However, their different structural roles in the market economy, coupled with their equally different—and unbalanced—roles in the household economy, mean that men and women face different constraints, options, incentives, and needs.

## Gender in the Market Economy

The relative contributions of men and women to the market economy (GDP) vary according to the national wealth, custom, and law. Generally speaking, where agricultural production is largely manual, women perform the bulk of the work. On the other hand, with a few exceptions, such as textiles (garment production), the majority of employees in most manufacturing businesses are men, as is the case in extractive industries and construction. Formal employment opportunities tend to be greater for men, especially for jobs that require travel, because women tend to be more tied to domestic duties. By contrast, women tend to be more active in the informal economy. However, this phenomenon has less to do with choice and more to do with women's efforts to support their families when formal employment opportunities are limited or do not allow the flexibility that informal employment permits.

One way to capture the dynamics of the varied contributions of men and women to the productive economy is in the "gender intensity of production" in different sectors. For example, in Uganda men and women are not equally distributed across the productive economy: agriculture is a female-intensive sector of production, whereas industry and services are male-intensive sectors (table 8.1).

In the formal sector men are also very much in the majority in senior positions. To some extent this dominance owes to the much greater time constraints of married women; these constraints limit their options and flexibility to respond to changing economic opportunities.

Frequently, an employer's attitude toward employing women is shaped by the fact that women of childbearing age can become pregnant. They require time off and, when they do have children, they have on occasion also to take time off to attend to family matters (sick family members, schooling, and so on). Hence, some employers prefer to employ men and older women, and to avoid younger women, in positions in which experience is important and work pressure is intense.

**Table 8.1**  Uganda: Structure of the Productive Economy

|  |  |  | Gender intensity of production | |
| --- | --- | --- | --- | --- |
| Sector | Share of GDP (%) | Share of exports (%) | Women (%) | Men (%) |
| Agriculture | 49.0 | 99.0 | 75.0 | 25.0 |
|   Food crops | 33.0 |  | 80.0 | 20.0 |
|   Traditional exports | 3.5 | 75.0 | 60.0 | 40.0 |
|   NTAEs | 1.0 | 24.0 | 80.0 | 20.0 |
| Industry | 14.4 | 1.0 | 15.0 | 85.0 |
|   Manufacturing | 6.8 |  | n.a. | n.a. |
| Services | 36.6 | 0.0 | 32.0 | 68.0 |
| Total | 100.0 | 100.0 |  |  |
| **Contribution to GDP** |  |  | **50.6** | **49.4** |

*Source:* Adapted from Elson, Evers, and Gideon 1998.
NTAEs = nontraditional agricultural exports; n.a. = not available.

On the other hand, in many factories in developing economies (garment production is a good example) women are favored as a cheap source of labor. Indeed, except in countries where the law stipulates equal pay, such as in the European Union, women are usually less well paid than men.[11] The pay gap is gradually closing, but if and when equality in employment terms is achieved, women are likely to remain unequal at home.

## Gender in the Household Economy

Nowhere is gender imbalance more marked than in the domestic household. Women and children are more vulnerable because tradition gives them less decision-making power and less control over assets than men, while at the same time their opportunities to engage in remunerative activities, and therefore to acquire their own assets, are more limited. Of course, there are single male parents and there are caring male partners who do their fair share, but it is normally the case that the burden of running the household economy falls principally on women. Among the major duties that they typically have to perform are child feeding and nurturing, provisioning and preparing food, cleaning, fetching fuel and water, and attending to sick relatives. These tasks are unpaid and nonmonetized.

Because much of their work goes unrecorded, women actually work more hours than men do. Figure 8.2 illustrates the disproportionate shares of hours worked by men and women in Benin.

Despite their huge unpaid contribution at home, women are still disadvantaged in terms of resource allocation within the household economy. Men tend to decide what proportion of their income they will retain for themselves and how much they will contribute to the household. In poor economies, women are often left to provide for the family and, in doing so, deny themselves the nutrition and health care a mother or expectant mother needs. This is especially true of antenatal care, with consequent increased risk of birth complications. When a mother is sick every family member is adversely affected.

Unfortunately, the family scenario is not always a happy one, especially for female members. They may face two additional hazards: gender-based violence and female genital mutilation.

### Gender-Based Violence

Because it often occurs in private and sufferers are intimidated (by fear or embarrassment), domestic violence is widespread and underreported. For

**Figure 8.2** *The "Double Workday" of Women in Benin*

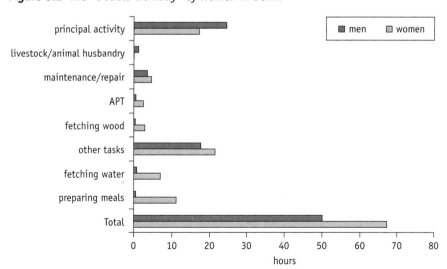

*Source:* UNDP 1998.
APT = agricultural produce transformation.

example, a study of Arabic and Islamic countries found that in four countries where reliable data were gathered at least one in three women is beaten by her husband (Douki and others 2003). Domestic violence constitutes a serious public health problem and is a major contributor to psychiatric symptomatology in women in both the developed and developing worlds (Douki and others 2003). Domestic violence affects women physically and emotionally, and it increases the risk of complications for expectant mothers. The Egyptian Demographic and Health Survey of 1995, to which a random national sample of 14,779 women responded, indicated that one of three Egyptian women ever married has been beaten at least once during marriage; one-third of those were abused during pregnancy (El Zanaty and others 1996).

The home is not the only place where women may be subjected to violence. The risk of violence toward women is prevalent in many societies. Girls and women who have to walk for several hours a day to collect firewood and water, or to go to and from school, are vulnerable to harassment and rape. And it is not only women undertaking domestic tasks who face such risks: those who are in lower-paid professions in which they are subject to male dominance (prostitution, for example) are also in danger. In Cambodia, gang rape is reportedly on the rise. The consequences of these violations for women's health, especially in terms of unwanted pregnancies and sexually transmitted infections (STIs), including HIV, are obvious.

## Female Genital Mutilation/Cutting

Another form of gender abuse is female genital mutilation/cutting (FGM/C).[12] This abuse refers to practices that involve cutting away part or all of a girl's external genitalia. Between 100 million and 130 million girls and women now alive in at least 28 African countries and two countries in the Middle East are estimated to have undergone FGM/C (WHO 1997).

FGM/C represents a fundamental violation of women's and girls' rights. It violates the rights to bodily integrity, to the highest attainable standard of health, and to be protected from harmful traditional practices, as well as to be free from violence, injury, abuse, torture, and cruel or inhumane and degrading treatment.

FGM/C is routinely traumatic. It is often performed under poor sanitary conditions by traditional practitioners. The immediate and long-term health consequences vary according to the procedure performed. Immediate complications include excruciating pain, shock, urine retention, ulceration of the genital regions, and injury to the adjacent tissues. Hemorrhage and infections can be of such magnitude as to cause death. Other complications include septicemia, infertility, and obstructed labor (WHO 1997), which of course have a direct effect on reproductive health.

FGM/C is no longer a practice to discuss: it must be stopped.

## Gender Imbalance and Poverty

Micro-level analyses reveal that gender-based asset inequality constrains growth and poverty reduction. Country case studies throughout Sub-Saharan Africa point to patterns of disadvantage that women, but not men, face in accessing the basic assets and resources needed to participate fully in realizing the region's growth potential. These gender-based differences affect supply response, resource allocation within the household, and, significantly, labor productivity. They have implications for the flexibility, responsiveness, and dynamism of African economies, and they limit growth (box 8.1).

The agricultural growth that Sub-Saharan Africa does not achieve because of gender inequality is not marginal to the continent's needs, because it affects food security and well-being, increases vulnerability, and further reinforces risk aversion. A case study in Burkina Faso shows how

---

**Box 8.1** *Gender and Growth: Missed Potential*

*Burkina Faso*: Shifting existing resources between the agricultural plots of women and those of men within the same household could increase output by 10–20 percent (see box 8.2).

*Kenya*: Giving women farmers the same level of agricultural inputs and education as men could increase yields obtained by women by more than 20 percent.

*Tanzania*: Reducing time burdens of women could increase household cash incomes for smallholder coffee and banana growers by 10 percent, labor productivity by 15 percent, and capital productivity by 44 percent.

*Zambia*: If women enjoyed the same overall degree of capital investment in agricultural inputs, including land, as their male counterparts, output could increase by up to 15 percent.

*Source*: Blackden and Bhanu 1999.

differences in access to key inputs, notably labor and fertilizer, lead to marked productivity differentials and differences in the supply responses of plots controlled by men and those controlled by women (box 8.2).

Parallel, comparative cross-regional macro data on gender differences in education and formal employment provide another basis for assessing the impact of gender inequality on growth. Over the 1960–92 period, Sub-Saharan

---

**Box 8.2** *Gender and Productivity in Burkina Faso*

In Burkina Faso, as elsewhere in Africa, different members of the household simultaneously cultivate the same crop on different plots. Detailed plot-level agronomic data provide striking evidence of inefficiencies in the allocation of factors of production across plots planted to the same crops but controlled by different members of the household. If two plots are identical in all respects except that one is controlled by the wife and the other by the husband, productive (Pareto) efficiency requires that yields and input allocations be identical on the two plots. The evidence shows that plots controlled by women have significantly lower yields than plots controlled by men. On average, yields are about 18 percent lower on women's plots. For sorghum, the decline is striking—about 40 percent. Even for vegetable crops in which women tend to specialize, the decline in yields is about 20 percent.

The econometric analysis shows that factors of production are not allocated efficiently across plots controlled by different members of the same household. Male labor, child labor, and nonhousehold labor are used more intensively on plots controlled by men. Plots controlled by women are farmed much less intensively than similar plots controlled by men. Although the diminishing marginal product of fertilizer is well documented, virtually all fertilizer is concentrated on the plots controlled by men. The gender yield differential is caused by the difference in the intensity with which measured inputs of labor, manure, and fertilizer are applied on plots controlled by men and women, rather than by differences in the efficiency with which these inputs are used. The production function estimates imply that reallocating actually used factors of production between plots controlled by men and those controlled by women in the same household could increase output by 10 to 20 percent. Household output could therefore be increased by the simple expedient of moving some fertilizer from male-controlled plots to similar but female-controlled plots planted in the same crop.

This evidence confirms a key point about intrahousehold relations in Burkina Faso, namely that men and women operate in a system of production in which some resources are neither pooled nor traded among household members. Allocative inefficiency, along with diminished output, is the result.

*Source:* Blackden and Bhanu 1999.

Africa, together with South Asia, had the worst initial conditions for female education and employment, and the worst record for changes in the past 30 years. The average number of total years of schooling for the female adult population in 1960 was 1.1 years. Gender inequality in schooling in 1960 was also very high in Sub-Saharan Africa: women had barely half the schooling of men. Females in the region have experienced the lowest average annual growth in total years of schooling between 1960 and 1992 (an annual increase of 0.04 years, raising the adult female population's average years of schooling by a mere 1.2 years). Females experienced a slower expansion in the growth of total years of schooling than males, and they have a weak position in formal sector employment. In 1970 the female-male ratio of formal sector employment was among the lowest in the developing world, and the share of female formal sector employment increased by only 1.6 percentage points between 1970 and 1990.

On the basis of these trends, a comparison of Sub-Saharan Africa and East Asia indicates that gender inequality in education and employment is estimated to have reduced the former region's per capita growth in the 1960–92 period by 0.8 percentage points per year. Moreover, gender inequality appears to account for up to one-fifth of the difference in the growth performance of Sub-Saharan Africa and that of East Asia. Although far from the overriding factor, gender inequality is an important contributor to Sub-Saharan Africa's poor economic performance.

## Interdependence of Market and Household Economies

Analysis of the time allocation of men and women captures the interdependence of "market" and "household" economies. As is well documented, women work longer hours than men because so much of women's productive work is unrecorded and not included in the System of National Accounts (SNA). For example, it is estimated that the SNA fails to capture nearly 60 percent of female activities in Kenya, compared with only 24 percent of male activities (Blackden and Bhanu 1999).

Children are closely integrated into household production systems, and the patterns that disadvantage female children begin very early. Poor households need their children's labor, sometimes in ways that also disadvantage boys. Domestic chores, notably fetching water and fuel, are one of the key factors limiting girls' access to schooling.[13]

The transport sector strikingly illustrates the interdependence between market and household economies and the associated time problem for

women. The gender division of labor leaves women with a far more substantial transport task in rural areas. Village transport surveys in Ghana and
Tanzania show that women spend nearly three times more time in transport
activities than men, and they transport about four times more volume
(Blackden and Bhanu 1999).

The interdependence of market and household economies results in
short-term intersectoral and intergenerational trade-offs within poor asset-
and labor-constrained households. These trade-offs suggest that investment
in the household economy would benefit the market economy in terms of
improved efficiency and productivity and, hence, growth. The trade-offs are
compounded by intrahousehold inequality and the complexities of intrahousehold relations. Examples of short-term trade-offs are those between

- different productive activities (labor allocation for food and cash crop
  production, especially where seasonal labor and cropping pattern
  constraints exist);
- market tasks and household tasks, for which rigidity in labor allocation for domestic tasks, lack of mobility, and time constraints limit
  response capacity; and
- short-term economic and household needs and long-term investment
  in future capacity and human capital (for example, fetching water
  [girls] and herding livestock [boys] limit households' options for
  sending children to school and breaking the intergenerational transmission of poverty).

Sectoral growth policies and priorities need to take account of these short-
term trade-offs and the positive externalities. Aligning the school year with
the cropping cycle, for example, can mitigate trade-offs at the household
level. Investing in the household economy and domestic labor-saving technology improves labor productivity and constitutes a positive externality for
the market economy. Most important, these trade-offs and externalities rein-
force the need to tackle the labor time constraints facing women and girls.

## Improving Health and Reducing Poverty
## by Narrowing the Gender Divide

Four public policy interventions could narrow the gender divide and contribute to improved health and reduced poverty. The first and most important
intervention is investment in girls' education. The second is concurrent
investments in the household economy, which are necessary if the full bene-

fits of investment in female education are to be realized. The third intervention is investment in basic and reproductive health—also necessary to realize the full benefit of female education investment. The fourth intervention is corrections to reduce the widely documented gender-based disparity in access to assets. Extensive micro-level data and case studies, along with emerging macroeconomic analysis, show systematically how gender differences in access to and control of these assets directly limit economic growth, and how gender inequality is therefore costly to economic and social development.

The priority given to specific actions within these interventions will vary according to different country circumstances. But to make progress, it will be necessary to encourage more open discussion about the relative roles of men and women to ensure widespread participation in and the formulation of inclusive policies and programs.

To conclude, strategies that build on an understanding of the links and synergies among poverty, gender inequality, and health will make an effective contribution to improving health outcomes, and to poverty reduction more generally, at both household and national levels.

# 9

## *Poverty and Reproductive Health*

An amazing volume of empirical work in the last five years has focused attention on the plight of the poor in the health sector. In 1999 a group of World Bank staff working on the relationship between health and poverty began publishing a series of country reports that highlighted persistent inequality in health outcomes and health system outputs in the more than 40 low- and middle-income countries (Gwatkin and others 2000). This exercise took advantage of a recently developed methodology that allowed researchers to infer relative wealth using readily available survey questions about asset ownership (Filmer and Pritchet 2001). The new technique for classifying wealth was used in the USAID-financed Demographic and Health Surveys (DHS).

Nobody should be surprised that the poor suffer more than the rich in terms of mortality, fertility, malnutrition, and morbidity, but the size of the gap between the rich and the poor has commanded the attention of policy makers and development agencies. As figure 9.1 shows, the gap in infant mortality rate (IMR) is consistently large in every region where data are available. The gap between the rich and the poor is evident not only in measures such as IMR and under-five mortality; it extends to measures of malnutrition, such as stunting and micronutrient deficiencies, as fertility outcomes.

As discussed in chapter 7, household factors and community influences play a large role in the production of good or bad health status. Because poverty is mainly a household and community characteristic, it is not surprising that the poor suffer most. They have less access to education, knowledge,

**Figure 9.1** *Rich/Poor Differences in Infant Mortality Rates in 56 Low- and Middle-Income Countries*

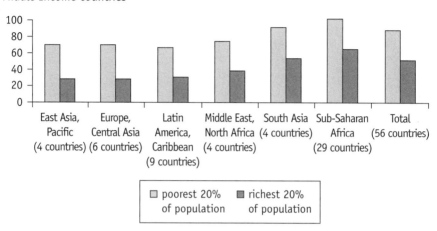

*Source:* World Bank 2005.

and resources. They have higher risk factors in terms of susceptibility to communicable diseases. They are strongly influenced by cultural factors or strict religious beliefs. They are the hardest to reach in terms of behavior change communication strategies. Given gender disparities (discussed in chapter 8), poor women are most at risk in the area of health, population, and nutrition.

## Not a Pretty Picture

The poor are more at risk than the rich and, as figure 9.1 shows, risks are usually realized; hence, mortality rates are higher for the most vulnerable in society. Both disappointing and surprising is how health sectors have failed to adjust to the larger needs of the poor. Moreover, the rich, not the poor, capture the larger share of the government subsidy for the health sector.

Analysis of the DHS for 56 low- and middle-income countries reveals deep and persistent inequalities in the use of health services. Figure 9.2 illustrates use of basic maternal and child health services by the rich and poor in the 56 low- and middle-income countries where the data are available. Figure 9.2a shows the coverage/use levels for the richest and poorest quintiles for antenatal care, oral rehydration therapy, immunization, attended delivery, treatment of fever, and women's use of modern contraception. The poor use considerably less of each of these basic maternal and health services than the rich.

***Figure 9.2*** *Use of Basic Maternal and Child Health Services in 56 Low- and Middle-Income Countries*

a. coverage rates for poorest and richest quintiles

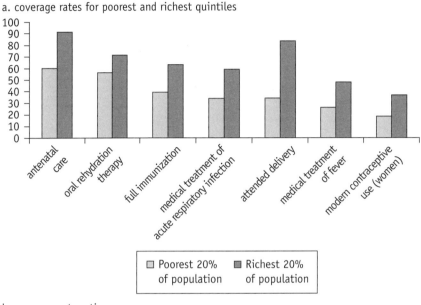

b. coverage rate ratios

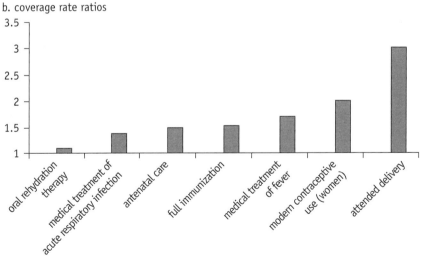

*Source:* World Bank 2005.

Figure 9.2b presents the same data as figure 9.2a but in a different format. Instead of showing utilization rates by group, the figure presents the odds ratio for service use by rich and poor quintiles. In other words, it represents the likelihood that a rich, rather than a poor, person uses the services. This format reveals where the rich-poor gap is the largest. The evidence indicates that not only are health sectors failing poor people in many countries but that the largest failure is in serving poor women. A woman from the richest quintile (20 percent of the population of a country) is *two times* as likely to use modern contraception than a poor woman and *three times* as likely to have an attended delivery.

## Who Benefits?

The utilization analysis presented above suggests that any assumptions made about health services serving poor people are probably false in many countries. And although distribution-friendly utilization analyses are powerful tools, they do not capture overall system subsidies very well, because services as public subsidies and budget allocations are not equally distributed across services and levels of care.

A tool that can capture all public subsidies to health and that is becoming increasingly popular is benefit incidence analysis (BIA). BIA is a crude but politically powerful way to identify the groups that are gaining from government spending. By simply combining two empirical facts—the identity of service users and the cost to the government of making the services available—it is easy to see which groups are benefiting the most from publicly provided or financed health services.

The problem with BIA is that it is data intensive. Two types of information are needed. The first is a detailed household survey that includes information on health services use (preferably by level of care) and that allows for grouping of individuals by socioeconomic characteristics (such as wealth or residence). The second type of information needed is the unit cost to the government of providing different types of services (typically a hospital overnight stay or an outpatient consultation at different levels of facilities).

With these two types of information, winners and losers can be identified in five steps:

1. Identify group users by socioeconomic category (income, sex, residence, tribe or caste, and so on).
2. Determine service use by group.
3. Calculate the unit cost for the service.

4. Subtract the out-of-pocket fees from cost.
5. Multiply the net unit cost by the group service use to determine group benefit.

A review of all BIA efforts in the health sector was put together a couple of years ago as part of the input for the *World Development Report 2004: Making Services Work for Poor People* (Filmer 2003; World Bank 2003). Analysis of data from 21 countries revealed that the overwhelming majority of health ministry budgets were more likely to serve the richest 20 percent than the poorest 20 percent of the population. The strongly negative finding held true even when only primary care budgets were reviewed.

Figure 9.3 and table 9.1 reflect the results of a BIA conducted in India. An examination of overall public spending on health in India (figure 9.3) reveals that despite repeated policy statements that the health sector is meant to serve the poor, only 10 percent of the government subsidy in health is captured by the poorest 20 percent in India; the richest quintile capture more than 33 percent of the health sector subsidy. Table 9.1 shows large variations across the different states in India. Kerala is the only state with pro-poor subsidies in health (as measured by the concentration index).

Another example of BIA use is the safe motherhood program in Vietnam. Researchers wished to measure how public subsidies for facility-based deliveries and antenatal care are distributed to different income groups across five levels of care. Table 9.2 shows the results for the richest and poorest quintiles and the five levels of care. The poorest quintile benefited more than the richest quintile at lower levels of care (commune health center and

**Figure 9.3** *Beneficiaries of Public Health Subsidies in India, 1996*

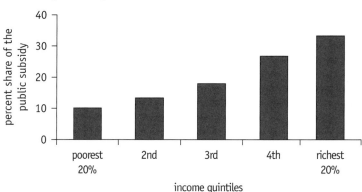

*Source:* Peters and others 2002.

**Table 9.1** *State-Level Inequalities in Health*

| Rank | State | Concentration index | Ratio of curative care subsidy to richest versus poorest quintile |
|------|-------|--------------------|-----------------------------------------------------------------|
| 1 | Kerala | −0.041 | 1.10 |
| 2 | Gujarat | 0.001 | 1.14 |
| 3 | Tamil Nadu | 0.059 | 1.46 |
| 4 | Maharashtra | 0.060 | 1.21 |
| 5 | Punjab | 0.102 | 2.93 |
| 6 | Andhra Pradesh | 0.116 | 1.85 |
| 7 | West Bengal | 0.157 | 2.73 |
| 8 | Haryana | 0.201 | 2.98 |
| 9 | Karnataka | 0.208 | 3.59 |
| | **All India** | **0.214** | **3.28** |
| 10 | North East | 0.220 | 3.16 |
| 11 | Orissa | 0.282 | 4.87 |
| 12 | Madhya Pradesh | 0.292 | 4.16 |
| 13 | Uttar Pradesh | 0.304 | 4.09 |
| 14 | Rajasthan | 0.334 | 4.95 |
| 15 | Bihar | 0.419 | 10.3 |

*Source:* Peters and others 2002.

**Table 9.2** *Distribution of Public Subsidies for Facility-Based Deliveries and Antenatal Care in Vietnam*
in Vietnam dong

| | Poorest 20% | Richest 20% |
|--|-------------|-------------|
| Central hospital | 116 | 437 |
| Provincial hospital | 91 | 562 |
| District hospital | 80 | 216 |
| Polyclinic | 78 | 40 |
| Commune health center | 360 | 338 |
| Total benefit | 726 | 1593 |

*Source:* Knowles 2000.

polyclinic), but the richest benefited more than the poorest at the highest, and most expensive, levels of care. The benefit to the richest women was more than two and a half times that to the poorest women.

## There Is Hope

The evidence presented in this chapter does not paint a positive picture of the ability or interest of health ministries around the world in serving poor people. So many factors may be working against the poor that any attempt to reach them with services will fail. A recent research effort is beginning to document cases in which concerted efforts to reach the poor have proven to be successful (Gwatkin, Wagstaff, and Yazbeck 2005). The Reaching the Poor Program has collected evidence from pilots, projects, and programs in Africa, Asia, and Latin America that have either proven to be pro-poor or have significantly improved the distribution of services and subsidies. Examples of success include

- expanding health insurance reach for the poor in Colombia,
- establishing community-based micro health insurance in Rwanda,
- contracting for primary health care with NGOs with incentives for reaching the poor in Cambodia,
- strengthening community ownership of service delivery through social funds in Latin America,
- increasing demand for basic services through conditional cash transfers for the poor in Mexico,
- implementing community-driven planning for reproductive health services for adolescents in Nepal,
- social marketing for antimalaria bed nets in Tanzania,
- improving the targeting of public subsidies within universal programs through geographic targeting of new investment in Brazil,
- cushioning the effects of user fees through a cost-recovery fund at hospitals in Cambodia,
- implementing community-based services by a local women's union in India (SEWA Union), and
- cushioning the effects of the financial crisis in Indonesia by using targeted health cards.

Given that the roots and manifestations of poverty vary from country to country and within large countries, a single approach is not the answer to addressing inequalities in health service use. Different approaches can be developed and implemented to address these inequalities. That said, successful programs share several characteristics. They have made reaching the poor an explicit goal and recognized the importance of analyzing the constraints faced by the poor and existing in health systems. Successful programs have also monitored service distribution and experimented with creative approaches to planning and delivering services.

# 10

## *Improving the Relevance of Health Services*

The Program of Action adopted by the 1994 International Conference on Population and Development represented a major departure from previous thinking on population and development. The ICPD moved the focus of the international population community beyond numbers of people and demographic targets and called for investments in people and in their health and education as the key to economic growth and sustainable development.

The ICPD endorsed a reproductive health approach to service delivery that addresses individuals' unmet reproductive health needs throughout their lives. RH services typically include treatment of reproductive tract infections, prevention and management of sexually transmitted diseases (including HIV/AIDS), maternity care, and family planning. Program managers are striving to understand and apply the new approaches and are seeking practical guidance on what to do and how to do it in their own countries.

One of the challenges facing health managers is implementing the reproductive health approach while carrying out health sector reforms. The two activities are potentially complementary and mutually reinforcing. In fact, effectiveness of reproductive health service delivery can be an excellent measure of how well the entire health system is working. Nevertheless, design and implementation of both the reproductive health and reform agendas present possible areas of conflict, which arise from the way in which services were delivered before reform and in which transitional steps toward reform and integrated reproductive health services are being managed today.

A typical health reform program will support delivery of a package of preventive and primary care for control of communicable and noncommunicable diseases, promotion and maintenance of reproductive health throughout the life cycle, and early detection and management (including referral) of reproductive health problems when they cannot be addressed at lower levels of the system (Bitrán y Asociados 1998). Table 10.1 presents an illustrative service package with various services provided at different levels of the health system (from community outreach to the district hospital). This chapter focuses on the service delivery matrix and the process involved in establishing it.

Reproductive health services often constitute a significant part of service packages. Incorporating reproductive health in these packages may require integration of services (family planning, for example) that had been delivered through a freestanding or vertical program, as well as strengthening of referral and other support systems. For this reason, those who champion reproductive health should link what they recommend for inclusion in the service package with other services and work with others on the design of the whole package rather than on reproductive health alone. Reproductive health specialists will be working with a range of other stakeholders in this process (consumers, nurses and doctors, program planners and managers, budget officers, local and national politicians, grassroots groups, and donors, to name a few); as expected, they will have varying views and concerns about what should be included.

Many considerations will shape the content and design of service delivery packages in specific settings: the health needs of the population, the services required at various levels to meet those needs, resource availability, capacity to deliver services, and consumer demand. Those who come from a specific program area (family planning, immunization programs, control of sexually transmitted infections, and so on) that is being folded into the essential package may also worry that the "integrated" approach to service delivery will place excessive burdens on systems that are already stretched and further dilute service quality. Effective design of an essential package requires participatory needs assessment, technical judgments about service delivery strategies, and analyses of the costs and institutional/management capacity of the health system.

Design of a service delivery matrix starts with three related tasks: (1) describing the service delivery system (levels at which services can be delivered); (2) deciding what services will be delivered at each level and what kinds of problems and procedures will be referred to higher levels; and (3) using appropriate service standards and norms for each type of service or procedure to specify the facilities, equipment, medicines, supplies, and skills required for delivery of each type of service. Health care specialists

**Table 10.1** *Illustrative Service Package, Including Reproductive Health and Other Primary/Preventive Services*

| Intervention | Community/household (outreach workers) | Clinic (or lowest-level fixed site facility)[a] | Health center: (a) outpatient surgery only; (b) inpatient surgery | District hospital (referral services) |
|---|---|---|---|---|
| **Family planning** | Community counseling; distribution of condoms, oral contraceptives | Manage/refer problems; provide injectables | Manage/refer problems (a); IUDs, Norplant (a); Sterilization (b) | Infertility |
| **RTI control and management** | Information on safe sex; recognition of symptoms | Counseling; symptomatic screening; symptomatic treatment | Testing (a); full treatment of asymptomatic problems (a) | Diagnostic procedures; specialized treatment; HIV screening |
| **Ante- and postnatal care, normal deliveries, management of emergencies** | Register pregnancies; home deliveries; recognize problems and arrange transport | Antenatal checkups; TT vaccination; obstetric first aid; IV fluids, antibiotics | Basic obstetric care (b); emergency obstetric care (b); postabortion care (b) | Comprehensive emergency obstetric care; ectopic pregnancy |
| **Nutrition** | Identify, treat anemia; counsel pregnant women; Vitamin A, iron folate | Manage supplementation program | | |
| **Management of child illness** | Feeding advice; vitamin A; home treatment for fever/malaria/diarrhea; care seeking (early recognition and referral) | Assess and classify ORT and feeding for diarrhea; antibiotics for bacterial ARI; antimalarial drug for fever (in malaria areas) | Assess and classify cough, diarrhea, fever, nutritional status; treat cough, fever/malaria, diarrhea, blood in stool, ear problems (a); refer severe cases (b) | Manage severe cases |

*(continued)*

**Table 10.1** (continued)

| Intervention | Community/household (outreach workers) | Clinic (or lowest-level fixed site facility)[a] | Health center: (a) outpatient surgery only; (b) inpatient surgery | District hospital (referral services) |
|---|---|---|---|---|
| **Immunizations** | Maintain registers | Immunization (EPI plus) | | |
| **Disease control** | Water, sanitation; identify TB suspects and provide DOTS to cases; manage malaria cases | Identify TB suspects and provide DOTS to cases; manage malaria | Diagnose and treat cases (a); secondary drugs for malaria (a); manage drug complications (a) | Manage severe cases |
| **Curative care** | Treat cuts, bruises, fever, stomach aches | Antibiotics and other medications, IV fluids | Other surgery (b) | |

*Source:* Authors.

a. Services offered at lower levels would normally be offered at higher levels as well, when appropriate, and are not repeated in higher-level cells.

ARI = acute respiratory infection; DOTS = directly observed treatment short course; EPI = Expanded Progamme of Immunization; IUD = intrauterine device; ORT = oral rehydration therapy; RTI = reproductive tract infection; TT = tetanus toxiod.

typically lead this process in consultation with key stakeholders, including health care consumers. Once they have specified the types of services to be delivered at different levels and identified the inputs needed to deliver them, they must collaborate with economists and financial experts, who will help determine the cost implications of the proposed package.

Most countries will deliver preventive and primary care at levels that start with community outreach and extend up to and include the district hospital, but not all countries have the same configuration of service delivery points at intermediate levels. Therefore, the structure of the service delivery matrix will vary from country to country. Figure 10.1 depicts two possible structures.

The next issue to be addressed in designing the matrix is what services will be delivered at each level. Figure 10.2 shows an antenatal and delivery care system in which home deliveries and community-based antenatal care are an option, along with delivery at health centers that provide services for normal deliveries as well as basic obstetric care. More complex problems and procedures are referred to higher levels—the district hospital and a referral hospital (perhaps the teaching hospital at the country's national university in the capital).

A variety of considerations will determine what is done where: community preferences (for example, to deliver at home), availability of personnel and facilities or the capacity to train and deploy appropriate staff, availability and location of facilities, cost of delivering services, and resources and different levels at which to cover such costs. Many of these constraints may

**Figure 10.1** *Two Possible Structures for Service Delivery*

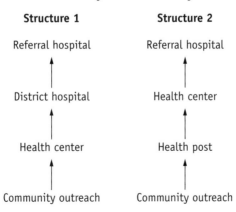

*Source:* Authors.

**Figure 10.2** *Antenatal and Delivery Care Services Defined by Level*

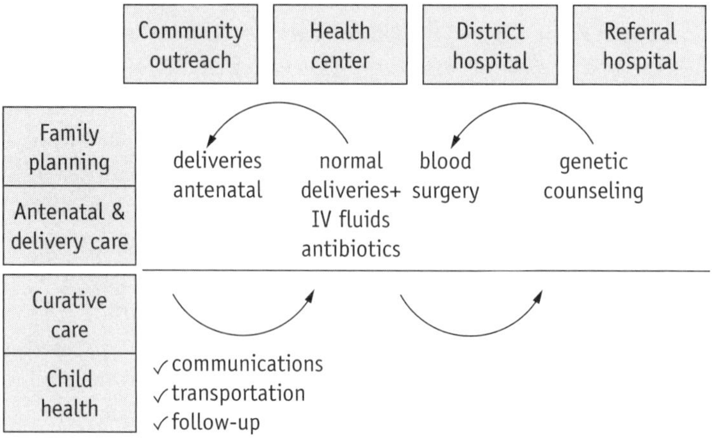

*Source:* Authors.

be fixed in the short run but could be changed over the longer run through planning and investments in health system development.

In addition to service delivery requirements at each level, attention must be given to what is needed to maintain an effective referral system (communications, transport, follow-up).

To deliver a given service at a given level, managers typically rely on service delivery norms set by the World Health Organization or professional associations representing practitioners in a particular realm of health care. With respect to delivery care, WHO has compiled guidelines for pregnancy, childbirth, and postpartum and newborn care (WHO 2003). These guidelines specify the type of each intervention or procedure, as well as the inputs (trained personnel, equipment and facilities, medicines and other consumables) required (figure 10.3). At the country level, these norms and requirements must be matched to in-the-field realities of existing health systems; proposals for services to be included in the package must be adjusted accordingly.

Poor countries may be delivering only a few of the services in the desired package. A major challenge is how to get from where the country is to where it wants to be, given existing resources and capacity as well as prospects for mobilizing additional resources and strengthening capacity. Priority setting will be required to plan a phased move from provision of the existing to the desired array of services. Key stakeholders in reproductive health and health reform need to find ways to work effectively with each other in this priority-setting process.

**Figure 10.3** *Standard Treatments and Inputs Specified by WHO for Antenatal and Delivery Care*

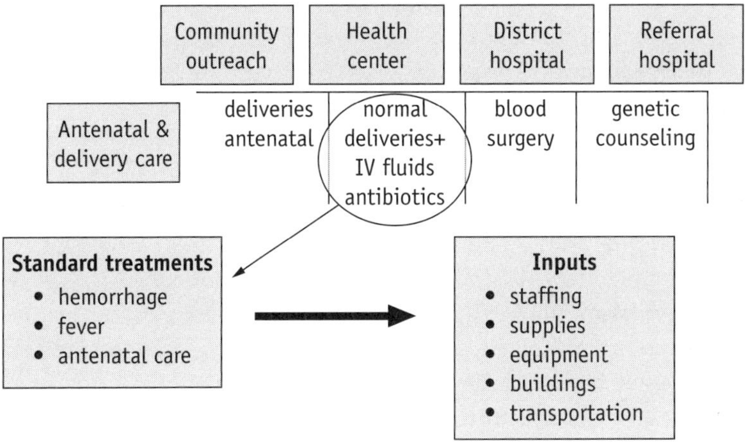

*Source:* Authors.

Assembling all of the information required to design the service package depicted in table 10.1 can be a long and sometimes contentious process, particularly if it is open to the views of consumers and other stakeholders who will bring nontechnical considerations to the table—for example, the custom of home deliveries. Ignoring such preferences (or failing to address them through effective health education) can lead to costly mistakes in the design of packages, which may look great to the experts but which offer services that are underutilized because there is no demand for them.

Once health experts have designed a package, they must deal with health economists, who will ask tough questions such as how much the package will cost (see chapter 11 on costing) and what services will be cut if the cost of the proposed package exceeds the amount of money available to finance it (see chapter 12 on prioritization).

The effort invested in producing the detailed service delivery matrix and specifying input requirements improves the bargaining position of health professionals in the dialogue with the economists, whose first reaction to a service package may be to consider it a collection of wish lists that the country cannot afford. The matrix enables health professionals to engage economists on details of input requirements, which is what the costing process is all about. As chapter 11 will show, costing is not rocket science, but it involves an enormous amount of attention to detail.

For a country to deliver a package of services (or to finance private providers to deliver it through a national insurance scheme), health professionals, economists, and other stakeholders will have to engage in dialogue and negotiations about the amount of services they each desire and the amount that financial and organizational resources will actually permit in the short run. Over the long run, the country may be able to increase investment by mobilizing more resources, improving the effectiveness of service delivery, and investing in human and physical capacity to deliver the package.

The transition will require restructuring and reorganization of service delivery and support systems, as well as resource mobilization and improved financing, which takes us back to the question of health reform. The reform effort should begin with a careful assessment of the health needs of the population and of the capacity of the existing system to meet those needs. It should then incrementally target investments to gaps in service capacity, support systems (including training), and management structures.

In many cases, critical reform decisions take little account of the real needs of the population or the realities of the country. A participatory effort is needed to formulate a service delivery package that addresses the needs of multiple stakeholders while also taking account of the limitations of budget, staffing, and infrastructure that often impede implementation of reforms (see chapter 14).

The service delivery matrix highlights non-clinic-based interventions as well as clinic-based activities, and, hence, it provides a more complete picture of the total program. The matrix also presents the connections among the various parts of the system in areas such as referrals and community participation.

# 11

## *How Much Does It Cost?*

Financial constraints motivate policy makers and service providers to make difficult decisions. If resources were abundant, prioritization would not be required, and consumers and service providers could consume and provide every good or service technically feasible. But even in the richest countries, resources are insufficient to provide every service. Financial constraints are much more binding in income-poor developing countries. In Nepal and Bangladesh, for example, the public sector spends less than $4 per person per year on all health and family welfare services; the situation is not much better in many poor countries in East Asia and Sub-Saharan Africa.

Not surprisingly, the cost question is on the lips of most policy makers, public health specialists, economists, donors/lenders, and ministry of finance decision makers. It has important implications and, surprisingly, many dimensions. Asked at different stages of the development of services or benefits packages, the question can take various forms:

- What are the available resources for proposed interventions?
- How much are we currently spending on these interventions?
- What is the unit cost of the interventions under consideration?
- What is the additional cost to provide these interventions?

The first question is typically asked by designers of a package of benefits or services at the outset of the development process. They request economists to examine the budgets for relevant agencies and analyze sources of funds (including private financing) as well as financial mechanisms, such as insurance, social security, or direct provision. Countries with established financial information systems for national health accounts are able to answer the first question quickly and without much effort and thereby determine the resource envelope for planning purposes.

The second question builds on the first by focusing on a particular set of interventions and the breakdown of expenditures into service-specific units. To answer it with some degree of accuracy, data from health and family welfare facilities are needed to help desegregate budget numbers. The level of required accuracy determines the techniques used and the data needs. Comparative data on relative spending among interventions allow advocates and policy makers to assess the balance (or lack thereof) within publicly provided or financed services.

The last two questions are at the heart of health package design. Most policy makers and public health specialists focus on the unit cost question. But economists insist that unit costs are irrelevant for policy decisions; for them, the important question is the additional cost question.

## Motivations for Asking Cost Questions

The first step in any costing activity is to clearly define the activity's objective. In many instances, the objective determines the methodology used and the data collected. Collecting and presenting information on costs and expenditures can serve advocacy, planning, implementation, or monitoring needs. A brief discussion of each follows.

### Advocacy

Costing spreadsheets for the World Health Organization's mother-baby health package illuminate the advocacy aspect of costing. The spreadsheets reflect a standard set of assumptions about a hypothetical rural district population. With minimal modification, base inputs can be used to obtain a rough estimation of cost based on "standard" treatment. The spreadsheets have been used to advocate for allocation of sufficient resources to the health sector and to compare the cost of the mother-baby package to the cost of other interventions.

### Planning

Cost and expenditure information plays an important role in development of operational plans. Many basic questions can be answered by examining the flow of public and private funds—for example, how much is being spent on the health sector, how much is expected to be available in the near future, what funding mechanisms are available, and what recurrent cost implications capital investments have. Activities such as public expenditure reviews, flow-of-funds analysis, national health accounting, recurrent costs analysis, and future resource projection can be integral inputs into planning.

Another activity important for planning is detailed costing of programs and interventions. This chapter examines the many dimensions of costing a package of population and reproductive health services and describes tools for managing costing activities.

### Implementation and Monitoring

Cost and expenditure information play an important role in implementing programs and in monitoring the inputs into the process. Well-designed financial information systems can improve the efficiency of the delivery system as well as the transparency needed for contracting and other procurement activities.

## The Costing Quality Checklist

Policy makers find it difficult to work with economists when it comes to costing health services. Their commonsense questions often meet with confusing answers. The Costing Quality Checklist (CQC) is designed to empower policy makers by helping them to understand the main dimensions of costing and to develop terms of reference for costing activities. The following is a short version of the CQC:

1. Are objectives clearly identified?
2. Does the selected methodology match the objectives with respect to choice of techniques, choice of approaches, and use of simulation models?
3. Does the methodology account for overhead or administrative costs?
4. Does the methodology correctly apportion joint costs?
5. Does the methodology distinguish between fixed and variable costs?
6. Does the methodology distinguish between recurrent and capital costs?
7. Does the methodology produce average or marginal costs?
8. Which point of view does the methodology take?

9. Does the methodology address opportunity cost or just accounting costs?
10. Does the costing exercise take advantage of all available data sources?
11. Are the data collection methods used appropriately?
12. Are all the assumptions clearly stated and realistic?
13. Were sensitivity analyses undertaken to test assumptions?

### Are Objectives Clearly Identified?

Clarity of objective, as noted above, is the starting point for ensuring quality and relevant outputs. If costing will be an input for prioritization, we would likely use a methodology that provides quick and somewhat crude estimates of the different elements of a package of services. If costing will be used to determine procurement needs in terms of drugs, equipment, labor, and construction, a more accurate methodology that is more time consuming and more resource intensive is required. Answering the first question of the CQC is the most important step in drafting the terms of reference for a costing exercise. Doing so will ensure that resources and methodologies are appropriate.

### Does the Methodology Selected Match the Objectives?

Most costing is nothing more than simple algebra. Two main approaches are top-down costing and bottom-up costing. In top-down costing of a package of health benefits or services, national or subnational budgets are disaggregated by type of service and level of care. In this two-step approach, the analyst first identifies all the resources in an aggregated budget that might be available for the proposed package of services. The analyst then allocates expenditures to levels of care delivery (different types of hospital and health facilities) and within these levels to the proposed health services.

Bottom-up costing takes the opposite tack. It starts with identification of all the service delivery elements of each level of care, then costs the inputs needed to deliver them, and finally aggregates the costs of all activities into a package cost estimate. This three-step approach builds up the cost estimates service by service and adds up all costs to reach a package estimate.

Each approach presents advantages and disadvantages (table 11.1), so determination of which one to use will depend on the objective of the exercise. If, for example, the objective is a detailed analysis of the cost elements of each service in order to establish a reimbursement schedule for an insurance

**Table 11.1** *Comparison of Top-Down and Bottom-Up Costing Approaches*

|  | Top-down | Bottom-up |
|---|---|---|
| **Level of detail** | Lower | Higher |
| **Accuracy (for each intervention)** | Lower | Higher |
| **Accuracy (for each package)** | Higher | Lower |
| **Completeness** | Better | May exclude elements |
| **Cost** | Cheaper | More expensive |
| **Time** | Faster | Longer |

*Source:* Authors.

system, a more accurate measure of costs for each intervention is needed and a bottom-up approach may be preferred, even if more expensive and time consuming. Other important determinants of the choice of methodology are the time available for the exercise, the data available, and the level of resources committed.

For most of the remaining questions of the CQC, the three basic steps of costing—identification, quantification, and valuation—should be kept in mind:

- Identification is the process by which all relevant inputs into the provision of a service are identified and classified. This step may appear to be the simplest in the process, but it is where many mistakes are made and where many mistakes can be avoided.
- Quantification is assigning nonmonetary quantities (natural units) to measure the contribution of inputs into the provision of the service to be costed. At this stage, the time a doctor spends on a service or the number of consumables used or drugs prescribed is counted.
- Valuation is assigning monetary value to the inputs quantified in the previous step.

### Does the Methodology Account for Overhead or Administrative (Indirect) Costs?

A simpler way of asking this question is "are we counting everything?" The question allows the policy maker to check up on the thoroughness of the economist or accountant working on the costing exercise and on the completeness of the product. Direct costs usually refer to resources directly identified with a health service or product. Examples of direct costs include salaries, contraception, and equipment. Indirect costs refer to resources needed to support service delivery but not directly identified with the service or the product. Examples include administrative costs and monitoring and evaluation costs.

At the identification stage of costing, the analyst must ensure that all possible indirect costs are reflected. Typical omissions include training (initial and refresher, training of trainers, orientation), overhead for training institutions, supervision costs, and administrative overhead.

At the quantification stage, the analyst must review how overhead costs are allocated to different services (see joint costs discussion below).

### Does the Methodology Correctly Apportion Joint Costs?

Some cost items, such as drugs and dedicated equipment, are used only for one type of intervention, while others, such as doctors and facilities, are used for a series of interventions. Nonjoint costs refer to resources that are used for one intervention. Examples include the cost of an intrauterine device, the cost of medicines, and the cost of disposable medical supplies. Joint costs refer to resources used for more than one intervention. Examples include costs of clinic resources, salaries, and equipment. Shared cost items should be divided among the different interventions in commonsense and practical ways.

At the identification stage of costing, the analyst must ensure that cost items are correctly identified as joint or nonjoint. At the quantification stage, the analyst must ensure that correct techniques (or commonsense rules of thumb) are used for allocation of joint costs.

### Does the Methodology Distinguish between Fixed and Variable Costs?

The main issue here is that some cost items grow with added applications of interventions, whereas others, like rent, are not a function of the number of patients or clients. The budgetary implications are important if utilization rates are expected to change. Fixed costs refer to inputs that do not vary with the quantity of output in the short run (about one year). Examples include rent, lease payments, and fixed salaries. Variable costs refer to inputs that vary with the level of outputs. Examples include supplies, food, and drugs.

At the identification stage of costing, the analyst must ensure that cost items are correctly identified as fixed or variable. At the quantification stage, the analyst must ensure that reasonable assumptions are made about expected output changes (see the discussion on simulations below).

### Does the Methodology Distinguish between Recurrent and Capital Costs?

Building a hospital is considerably different from buying consumables in that the hospital can be used for a long period of time, whereas consumables lose their value after use. Recurrent costs are resources associated with inputs that will be consumed or replaced in one year or less. Examples include salaries, maintenance, and medicines. Capital costs are resources that have a life expectancy of more than one year. Examples include buildings and machines. Because of the time dimension, a dollar spent on building a hospital or buying a piece of equipment should not be accounted for in the same way as a dollar spent on drugs.

At the identification stage of costing, the analyst must ensure that each cost item is clearly identified as recurrent or capital. At the quantification stage, the analyst must identify the expected number of years of operation for capital cost items. At the valuation stage, the analyst must ensure that appropriate annualization rules are used in costing capital costs and must check on the valuation given when market prices are unavailable.

### Does the Methodology Produce Average or Marginal Costs?

This question is the slipperiest on the CQC. Average cost is the total cost divided by the number of units of output. Examples include the average cost of a visit to a clinic or the average cost of an overnight stay at a hospital. Marginal cost is the extra cost of one additional unit of output. An example is the cost of expanding coverage of an existing service or intervention.

Choosing an average or marginal cost focus depends on the objective of the costing exercise. If the objective is to examine variations across levels of delivery or regions, average costs are more important. If expanded delivery is under consideration, marginal costs are more important.

### Which Point of View Does the Methodology Take?

The issue here is accounting for costs borne by a community but not by the government or providers. This issue is important when considering benefits or services targeted at the poor, because one of the important determinants of service use is the cost of transport and the ease of physical access. Perspectives can be provided by the ministry of health (program costs), other government entities (transfers such as workers' compensation), consumers (user costs such as transportation costs and waiting time), and insurance providers.

At the identification and quantification stages of costing, the analyst must ensure that all identified costs are consistent with the costing perspective.

### Does the Methodology Address Opportunity Cost or Just Accounting Costs?

Opportunity cost is a rarely accounted for cost item in health sector cost studies but a critical factor for most commercial businesses. Because any expenses incurred to provide a service could have been used instead to earn a return (such as interest rates on savings accounts), the missed opportunity to earn a return should be counted as a cost. Accounting (financial) costs include all outlays made by the program to purchase goods and services. Opportunity (economic) costs include the value of the most productive alternative use of the resources.

### Are the Data Collection Methods Used Appropriately?

At the heart of costing is data collection. By looking closely at the data sources and the methods that were used to collect data, policy makers can ensure that data are reliable and representative.

Cost data are needed for labor (salaries and benefits); medications, contraceptives, and vaccines; supplies; training (inservice, preservice), operation and monitoring; supervision and monitoring; equipment; vehicles (transportation costs); buildings; and information campaigns.

Data sources and data collection methods include ministerial accounts (ministry of health), provider or facility records, donor/lender records, facility-based surveys (time-use surveys, equipment and supplies surveys, and utilization surveys), household surveys, insurance records, market surveys for prices, solicitation of expert opinion, health management information systems (demographic and epidemiological information), central purchasing organizations, and essential drugs programs.

### Are All the Assumptions Clearly Stated and Realistic?

All the needed cost data are rarely available, therefore cost exercises should list all the assumptions made and provide the rationale for making them.

Three basic questions need to be asked. Are the assumptions made explicit and clearly stated? Are the assumptions realistic? Were simulations undertaken to test assumptions and identify cost implications?

### Were Sensitivity Analyses Undertaken to Test Assumptions?

Listing and defending assumptions are insufficient. Policy makers need to know if assumptions are important enough to make a sizable difference in the final estimates of cost. Testing the implications of assumptions by systematically changing them and reestimating the results is therefore important.

Simulation models help policy makers understand the cost implications of a variety of policy changes, such as alternative plans for phasing in interventions, different forms of targeting, alternative technical interventions, changes in delivery strategy, and institutional reforms. The models can be used to perform sensitivity analysis for testing assumptions, such as those about coverage rates and price changes (including exchange rate fluctuations).

# 12

## Prioritization in the Health Sector: A Guide for the Perplexed

Every year health ministries develop annual budgets for the health sector. Every year donors, academicians, advocacy groups, medical trade unions and professional organizations, and health service managers and providers complain that the budgets have the wrong priorities. Although these groups are united in their unhappiness with the priorities reflected in these budgets, they disagree on what the priorities should be and on how the prioritization process should be conducted.

A review of the literature reveals the lack of consensus in the policy and academic communities on how best to prioritize health sector budgets. What it does not reveal is how countries actually prioritize health expenditures.

The objective of this chapter is to empower reproductive health champions by introducing them to the players in the health budgeting process, their objectives, the political realities that drive the process, and some techniques for evaluating priorities.

### Never Enough Money

Developing priorities within government budgets for the health sector is akin to the experience of a family struggling to live within a budget. Both activities face the same problem, which also happens to be the main driver of microeconomic theory—namely, limited resources and unlimited wants.

The two activities are similar in other ways:

- Prioritization is a highly political process in which the final result depends primarily on the relative position of power of the various advocates.
- The process will most probably produce clear winners and losers due to the difficulties in developing win-win solutions (there is simply not enough money). A standard result is some form of rationing.
- Failure to reach a final consensus leads to a situation in which those controlling the resources make the final decisions.

So how should policy makers, facing a resource constraint, make decisions about what to finance? As this chapter will show, there are no simple answers. Moreover, the different players involved in the health sector (see box 12.1 for an irreverent look[14]) bring different (and sometimes contradictory) objectives, decision criteria, and tools to prioritization.

## Selection Criteria

Left to its own devices, each advocacy group would use criteria tied to its objectives to set priorities.

### Equity Considerations

Equity means many things to many people. With respect to groups, it could involve income categorization, gender, age cohorts, tribes, social classes, or regional clusters. With respect to measures, equity can refer to health and family welfare outcomes, access to goods and services, or financial burden. Any number of definitions or dimensions of equity can be constructed. Advocates for equity will assign a higher value to services or goods that would more likely benefit the group for which they are advocating.

### Burden of Disease

Whether measured in disability-adjusted life years (DALY), quality-adjusted life years (QALY), or years of life lost, the burden of disease (BOD) uses a common currency (for the lack of a better term) to associate a comparable set of burden numbers to a list of health conditions. The numbers can be presented by order of burden and by population subgroup to provide useful information for different advocacy groups. For BOD to be useful in

**Box 12.1** *An Irreverent Look at Players and Objectives in the Health Budgeting Process*

In every prioritization exercise in the health budgeting process, you'll find topic-specific advocates who have clear objectives and who use data as strategically as they can to advance their objectives. Here's how to tell them apart.

 **Economists.** Also known as practitioners of the dismal science. Prefer not to be called "bean counters."

 *Objective:* Economists are driven by a singular need to clearly define the role of the state versus the roles of markets and the private sector. They will agree to include equity as an objective, but their primary interest is efficiency and optimal production and utilization of goods and services.

 *Tools:* The best tool available to economists in a prioritization exercise is the fact that almost nobody understands them. Concepts like *public goods, externalities,* and *risk pooling* tend to be particularly baffling to other advocates. To economists, government intervention should always be justified explicitly, government financing should always be highly selective, and government provision should be the tool of last resort.

 **Epidemiologists and public health specialists.** Especially known for their optimistic outlook on life.

 *Objective:* To obtain public resources for interventions targeting the main sources of the burden of disease (BOD). May use assumptions that would be called "sweeping," even by an economist.

 *Tools:* Sophisticated measures of the BOD[15] and universal measures of the cost effectiveness of a variety of interventions. Plus, they have really cool charts.

 **Politicians and administrators.** Also known as "clients." Often seen at ribbon-cutting ceremonies.

 *Objectives:* Politicians and administrators who will implement change are driven by a strong sense of political reality. They realize that that change (perceived or real) can bring political as well as technical risks, and can be seen as confirmation of their past actions, whether successful or not. They tend to prefer the status quo, and may not see private sector providers as friends to the degree that economists do.

 *Tools:* Since implementers are the owners of any intervention, who needs tools? But implementers can also claim (rightly or wrongly, depending on where) to be the true voice of the real client, the people.

*(continued)*

---

**Box 12.1**  *(continued)*

**Equity advocates.** May be known as "the politically correct."

*Objective:* To address long-standing imbalances in gender, family welfare, and health service access and outcomes for the poor. They like the word "empowerment." Their ability to frame the inequity issue is sharp; their proposed solutions, maybe not quite as sharp.

*Tools:* Pro-poor advocates have as an advantage the empirical fact of inequity in every health sector in the world. They use quantitative tools such as benefit incidence analysis or outcome incidence analysis to point to the problems, and qualitative tools such focus group work to point to possible answers. Gender equity advocates use the same tools as the pro-poor group but have the added advantage of being the only people able to talk about gender issues without sounding sexist.

**Health services providers.** Found on the front lines. Probably belong to trade unions.

*Objectives:* Individually, these providers may be interested in proposed reforms (as long as "reform" isn't just a code word for layoffs) and want to do good, but as group they are subject to union objectives, chief of which may be employment security and political clout.

*Tools:* The threat of walkouts or strikes is one very visible tool, but the political clout of their unions may be the more useful.

**Lenders and donors.** Also known as development partners. May be seen at prioritization meetings driving (or being driven) around in very large sport-utility vehicles.

*Objectives:* Sometimes difficult to grasp. Interested in reform and concerned about management.

*Tools:* Money.

---

prioritization, the analysis should be country specific, use recent data, and be based on a well-functioning and representative set of information systems. Otherwise it will be attacked as a misrepresentation of the true disease burden.

## Cost-effectiveness

Health specialists use cost-effectiveness to maximize positive health outcomes with available resources, but they shun a cousin of cost-effectiveness, cost benefit analysis, for assigning monetary value to human life. To be accurate, what is now called cost-effectiveness is actually cost utility, because the measure of effectiveness used (QALY or DALY) assumes preferences.[16]

### Public or Easily Shared Goods

The distinction between public and private goods is based on two characteristics of a good or service that affect the market's ability to provide a socially optimal quantity. These characteristics of a public good are consumption by multiple individuals or households at the same time (nonrival consumption) and inability to prevent that consumption (nonexclusionary provision). The overwhelming majority of health and family welfare services are private goods according to this definition. But public health specialists, who define their jobs as safeguarding the public health, find it difficult to accept this definition. Economists argue that pure public goods, such as the provision of public health information, should receive more public attention (and probably more public resources) than private goods.

### Externalities

Externalities refer to the costs and benefits of goods and services that are different for society than they are for the producers and consumers directly involved in the exchange.[17] Although health services are private in nature, they produce benefits to society beyond the direct benefits to the consumers. Because of that difference and without government action, markets will most likely produce goods and services with a strongly positive benefit externality at less than the socially optimal level. Economists argue that if positive externalities are large, public attention may be required, and in some cases public financing or even public provision is justified.

### Risk Pooling

Some health conditions are rare and too costly for most uninsured individuals to pay for out of pocket. Economists have identified some characteristics of health insurance markets—moral hazard and adverse selection—that will most likely make these markets fail without some element of public intervention. Therefore, economists would argue that public intervention to create insurance markets is justified on efficiency terms.

## Selection Criteria for Benefit or Service Packages

Packages of benefits or services became especially popular after publication of the World Bank's *World Development Report 1993: Investing in Health.* Selection of the benefits or services to be included in a package involves additional criteria.

### Existing Capacity to Deliver

Given resource constraints, the capacity of a system (public or private) to deliver proposed benefits or services should be considered. Advocates must understand not only current capacity but also take into account the investment costs of expanding services or adding new ones (interventions or benefits).

### Linkages across Services (Systems Approach)

A defining characteristic of a package is that many of its services are delivered at different levels of service. Package designers should consider the capacity of each level of service delivery as well as the linkages between levels.

### Budget Rigidities

Potential changes in how expenditures are directed are not always politically feasible. The two most difficult issues are service cuts and staffing changes that may be resisted by the upper-middle class and professional groups of service providers—two politically powerful constituencies.

### Transition Costs

Developing a package of services or benefits may involve changing the focus and orientation of service delivery or financing mechanisms. Costs associated with the transition can be large and need to be factored into the prioritization process.

## Prioritization Approaches

What makes prioritization especially challenging is that there are no clear rules to follow.[18] Four approaches are described below.[19] Each has advantages and disadvantages. Elements of each could be combined to tailor an approach appropriate for a specific country.

## Defining Categories of Care

In the early 1990s New Zealand's government broadly defined general categories of care. Politicians and health providers were left to make decisions about resource allocations within the categories. Although this approach limits political opposition, its lack of specificity may cause inefficient resource allocations and create conflicts of interest.

## Using Various Criteria to Select a Package of Services

The United Kingdom, the Netherlands, and the state of Oregon in the United States have provided or financed a basic package of services selected on the basis of criteria (such as those noted above) agreed on by the public sector. This approach produces a specific set of benefits, but implementing it is not easy because of the difficulty of achieving consensus on the relative weight assigned to each criterion.

## Using Cost-Effectiveness to Select a Package of Services

Other countries collect information on the costs of proposed interventions and use BOD or some other criterion to measure and compare the interventions' benefits. Social preferences can influence how the different benefits are combined and valued. This approach combines qualitative and quantitative methods, but it requires data at a level of detail typically not available. Moreover, it does not take into account the economic rationale for public intervention.

## Using Treatment Guidelines

Other countries focus on the efficacy of different interventions and provide guidelines for treatment to practitioners and patients. This approach identifies when services are medically beneficial but often reflects neither economic considerations nor community preferences and values.

# Who Loses?

Development of a benefits package inevitably produces losers (people who receive fewer benefits or services than others), especially in poor countries with large populations and small health budgets. This reality is referred to as "rationing."

No budget, or any other political document for that matter, will high-light the losers. But equity advocates have developed tools to identify the losers. Some of these tools were discussed in chapters 7 and 8 on gender and wealth inequality.

Groups that make the loudest noise about their perceived needs are likely to get the most resources. Those segments of society with the least "voice" or political influence—rural residents, the poor, and socially mar-ginalized groups—are likely to get the least resources, though their needs may be the greatest.

This assumption has been borne out by research on the equity dimension of public health spending. Two relatively crude approaches have been employed in this research. The first approach (described in chapter 8) exam-ines both supply-side information on expenditures and costs and informa-tion on the use of health services by different population groups. The second approach examines the supply side only—that is, identifies where public resources in the health sector flow.

Following the money is more easily said than done. Budgets are designed in ways that make detailed examination of progressively smaller allocations difficult. The main obstacle to deciphering a budget is budget heading codes. (For example, items accounted for under the health preven-tion and promotion heading are often surprising.) Cost headings cannot be taken at face value. More important is what health ministry accountants used to classify these headings.

Once budget heading codes have been cracked, answers to questions about the way resources are targeted will identify the losers. With respect to services, are resource flows addressing diseases of the poor?[20] Are they going to preventive health promotion? Behavior change communications? Appropriate levels of care delivery? With respect to geography, are resources flowing to regions with the most need? To rural areas or urban slums?

Research typically shows that rural areas and urban slums receive less public spending than other areas. Moreover, countries are spending less on interventions that address the needs of the poor at levels of care and facili-ties accessible by the poor.

# 13

## Influences Outside the Health Sector

Most maternal deaths and disabilities are preventable, and the interventions required to prevent them are known. So what are the barriers that keep women from utilizing interventions? Poor health sector performance is one reason: lack of trained personnel, poor deployment of personnel, ineffective referral, substandard treatment at referral centers, lack of suitably equipped ambulances, lack of medicines and equipment, and so on. Economists refer to them as supply-side barriers.

### Demand-Side Barriers

Economists also pay attention to demand-side factors that determine whether or not a mother utilizes appropriate preventive interventions, and, in the event of a life-threatening emergency, whether or not she and her family and community recognize and seek appropriate care. Demand-side barriers operate at the individual, household, and community levels, as outlined in table 13.1.

### Non-Health-Sector Barriers

Chapter 7 discussed the ways in which household behaviors and resources affect reproductive health outcomes. This chapter explores links at other levels: communities, other sectors and factors that affect or relate to the health system, and public policies and actions, as shown in figure 6.1.

**Table 13.1**  Demand-Side Barriers to Utilization of Health Care

| Barrier | Example |
| --- | --- |
| Information on health care choices/providers | Lack of knowledge of providers |
| Education | Little ability to assess health choices and negotiate access to appropriate providers |
| Indirect consumer costs | Long and slow travel to medical facilities; need for patient/caregiver to stop working for long periods in order to seek care |
| Household preferences | Asymmetric control over household resources |
| Community/cultural preferences, attitudes, and norms | Reluctance to seek care for women outside home; resistance to modern medical care to assist with delivery |
| Price/availability of substitute products and services | Seeking treatments from inappropriate providers |

*Source:* Ensor and Cooper 2004, p. 70.

Among the specific links and the ways in which they influence maternal health outcomes are

- community gender norms, which influence the capacity of women, particularly poor women, to access services;
- community readiness to mobilize resources (for example, credit and transport) to supplement government-sponsored services;
- attitudes toward gender-based violence, the adverse effects of which on maternal health outcomes are well documented;
- household, community, and societal guidelines on education— including any restrictions on the education of girls—that influence behavior and attitudes toward maternal health outcomes;
- household and community access to and supply of transport and communication critical for saving the lives of mothers who experience an obstetric emergency;
- employment terms that can deter pregnant women from taking time off to attend antenatal clinics and employment conditions that negatively affect the health of pregnant women and their unborn babies; and
- macroeconomic policies—for example tariffs and exchange rate policies—that can have a major impact on the costs of medicines, transport, and communications.

The focus of this chapter, however, is on interventions in sectors other than health and on public policies that affect specific reproductive health outcomes, particularly maternal and newborn survival.

## Community Factors

Community factors include both community values that shape household attitudes and behaviors and the physical and environmental conditions in the community. The community influences health outcomes principally through norms and values related to virginity, fertility, contraceptive use by youths, abortion, sexual education in schools, cultural practices such as female genital mutilation/cutting (FGM/C), and male dominance. In turn, these norms and values are influenced by religious, political, and social leaders and are spread through the community by the media and groups such as women's, youth, and nongovernmental organizations (NGOs); tribal leaders; and traditional healers, including traditional birth attendants and their organizations.

Factors that affect both health outcomes and the pace of change in a community include environmental factors, such as vehicles, roads, clean air, water supply, sewage systems, and types of local businesses (for example, beer and alcohol brewing in the community and the number and opening hours of bars).

## Related Sectors

Among other sectors and factors related to health outcomes, the most important are typically education, transport, energy, water and sanitation, nutrition, social conditions, employment, and the media.

### Education

Education of women influences reproductive health through a variety of channels, including childbearing attitudes, health-seeking behaviors, and earning opportunities. Early gains in female literacy played an important role in morbidity and mortality rates (MMR) declines in Malaysia and Sri Lanka (Pathmanathan 2003). In a review of linkages among women's education, autonomy, and reproductive behavior, Jejeebhoy (1995) noted that education enhances women's knowledge about the outside world and makes them more aware than uneducated women of the importance of family health and hygiene as well as the treatment and prevention of illness. It also gives women greater decision-making autonomy within the home. At the same time, Jejeebhoy cautioned that contextual factors influence the impact of education on women's participation in household decision making, so that participation is likely to be weaker in a society characterized by a high degree of gender stratification.

Focusing specifically on maternal mortality, McCarthy (1997) finds that women's education might affect maternal mortality by

- reducing numbers of pregnancies (and lifetime risk of complications) through later marriage and increased use of contraceptives;
- enabling women to be better informed about the importance of antenatal care, and the symptoms of complications, thereby increasing the likelihood that they will make more timely decisions to seek treatment;
- making women healthier and less likely to suffer complications;
- giving women better physical access to treatment facilities (because a higher proportion of educated women live in urban centers); and
- making women better off and more able to pay for care or be well treated by care providers because of their status.

None of these potential links guarantees that education will have the hypothesized impacts,[21] at least in the short term. However, there is little doubt as to the longer-term impact of education in influencing attitudes toward a range of factors that, in turn, determine health outcomes. Some of these factors are discussed below.

Education is closely linked to gender status and the ways in which gender stratification affects access to household resources and use of health care services (Kunst and Houweling 2001). Work on intrahousehold bargaining power in Indonesia (Beegle and others 2001) found that women who were more educated than their husbands were more likely to obtain antenatal care and, generally, that education enables a woman to make decisions regarding her reproductive health care. Education is also linked to several of the other factors that may enhance or limit access to lifesaving interventions. Research on the impact of cost recovery on use of services has shown that educated women are more likely to understand and use exemption schemes (Newbrander and others 2000), and the transport literature highlights the links between education and access to and use of transport to health facilities.

## Transportation

Delays in reaching a treatment facility pose life-threatening obstacles for women who experience an obstetric emergency. Such delays can be the result of physical accessibility factors such as distance to a facility; the availability, suitability, and cost of transport; and the condition of roads, all of which affect the time required to get a mother to a facility once the decision to seek care has been made (Thaddeus and Maine 1994). Many countries with high MMRs (Afghanistan, Pakistan, Nepal) also have large populations living in remote areas that have poor road links to facilities that can provide lifesaving interventions. In Zimbabwe, unavailability of transport is reported to have been a factor in 28 percent of deaths in a rural area that was studied (Fawcus and others 1996). In the case of hemorrhage, 50 percent of deaths were attributable to transport-related delays.

Though few road studies have focused specifically on health, and hardly any on maternal health, the available evidence suggests that transport is an important factor in the delays that threaten the lives of poor women. A review of health-seeking behavioral responses to cost recovery (Newbrander and others 2000) found that poor people in Tanzania traveled an average of over 60 kilometers for care, whereas the nonpoor traveled only 15 kilometers. There were similar findings in Kenya. The authors mention several possible reasons, including the likelihood that the nonpoor have their own transport and that the poor travel farther to attend a facility where fees would be waived. A review of obstacles to health care (Ensor and Cooper 2004) found studies reporting that transport accounts for 28 percent of all total patient costs in Burkina Faso, 25 percent in northeast Brazil, and 27 percent in the United Kingdom. In Bangladesh, transport was reported to be the second most expensive item for patients after medicines (CIET-Canada 2001). A participant in one of the focus groups in that study said, "The hospital is far away and it costs a lot to travel there. We can easily buy medicines from the village doctors with this money. We spend money to go to the hospital, but we don't even get medicines there, so why should we go to the hospital?"

Country-level poverty analyses conducted by the World Bank have shown that the quality of rural road networks is a factor in the social and economic isolation of the rural poor. Research on the impact of improved rural road networks has focused mainly on travel time. For example, a poverty assessment for Guatemala found that road closures were a major constraint on access to schools, work, and markets, and that households in the poorest income quintiles were much more affected (45 percent versus 12 percent) than the richest (World Bank 2003). Villagers identified giving birth as a risk because mothers could not reach health centers because of inadequate road access, particularly during the rainy season. Improved roads cut farm-to-market travel time from more than 10 hours to 1–2 hours. Although the research did not assess the impact on access to emergency obstetric care, these reductions in travel time have clear implications for reducing distance-related obstacles to timely management of emergencies. An earlier study of the impact of roads on access to services in Morocco found similar patterns. The road project contributed to clear gains in women's use of health services (World Bank 1996). Similar results were shown for girls' school attendance, which increased much more than boys' attendance: 40 percent versus 10 percent. Lack of roads posed a lesser obstacle for boys than for girls.

The quality and availability of roads is only one transport obstacle. The availability, type, and cost of transport is clearly another. Research conducted by African partners in the Prevention of Maternal Mortality Network found that poor roads, lack of vehicles, and high transport costs were major causes of delay in deciding to seek and in reaching emergency obstetric care (Samai and Sengeh 1997). That study reports the positive impact of efforts to improve transport and communication, along with community support and education activities, on the numbers of women getting treatment for obstetric emergencies, with consequent reductions in maternal deaths in the project area. Similar results have been reported for Nigeria (Essien and others 1997), Uganda (Lalonde and others 2003), and northwestern Tanzania (Ahluwalia 2003). These studies emphasize the role of community organizations in planning for and dealing with emergencies, including preparation of delivery plans, mobilization of resources through community funds, reduction of transport costs, and strengthening of the referral chain.

### Energy

Though not as pervasive as other barriers, lack of continuity of energy supply is nonetheless a factor in countries where load shedding is frequent. Hospital procedures can be halted and delayed if backup emergency power is not installed or is nonoperational. In rural areas without electricity, inadequate lighting and difficulty in sterilizing instruments adds to the risks in deliveries and abortions.

### Water and Sanitation

Provision of safe water has been cited as a factor in the declines of mortality in developed countries (van Poppel and van der Heijden 1997), and lack of sanitation and safe water, along with poor personal hygiene, are known to be major factors in the wide prevalence of parasitic diseases in poor countries. Studies of the impact of safe water on infant and childhood mortality typically do not focus separately on neonatal mortality, but they recognize that waterborne diseases can undermine the health of pregnant women, because they cause anemia, a risk factor for mothers as well as their newborns (Santiso 1997). A study in Africa (Paul 1993) cites unsafe water supply as well as pollutants from fuels used in cooking as risk factors in the high MMRs of the countries studied. In countries with MMRs under 30, 92 percent of households have safe water, compared with 51 percent in countries with MMRs over 1,000. The link between water supply and morbidity and neonatal mortality rates (NMRs) involves both household and community factors. A household's consumption of water may be constrained by prices, income, and other household variables, even if water is supplied at the community level. Jalan and Ravallion (2001) have observed that health gains largely bypassed poor children when piped water was available in their community, particularly when the mother was poorly educated.

## Nutrition

An adequate supply of the right foods is essential to avoid poor nutrition, another key factor in maternal and neonatal mortality. Because poor nutrition and closely spaced births are linked to maternal and neonatal mortality, nutrition deserves priority attention. Improved nutrition can help avert anemia, which is a high risk in the event of malaria during pregnancy. Poor nutrition among pregnant women contributes to high MMRs in many countries. In India anemia is an indirect factor in 64.4 percent of maternal deaths (Buckshee 1997). As the Safar Banu case demonstrated, gender stratification and attitudes also contribute to these deaths through household behaviors that deprive poor women of adequate nutrition, not only during pregnancy but also during their childhood and adolescence, which leads to small stature and higher risk of delivery complications.

## Social Conditions

Social conditions are dominant factors in influencing the behavior of individuals and communities. Housing that poor people can afford is more likely to be located near noise, pollution, and noxious social conditions. Blue-collar occupations tend to be more dangerous than white-collar occupations. Social networks with high-status peers are less likely to expose a person to secondhand smoke.

Socioeconomic resources shape many circumstances that affect health. These circumstances include access to the best doctors; knowledge of beneficial health procedures; friends and family who support healthy lifestyles; smoking cessation; getting flu shots; wearing seat belts; eating fruits and vegetables; exercising regularly; living in neighborhoods where garbage is picked up frequently, interiors are lead-free and asbestos-free, and streets are safe; having children who bring home useful health information from good schools; working in safe occupational circumstances; and taking restful vacations. It is not surprising, then, how critical a role social conditions play in the production of health outcomes (Link and Phelan 2002).

Improving social conditions is not so much about programs that make financial resources available to remedy poor conditions as about educating the population to want to achieve sustained improvement. For example, cleaning up streets to reduce unsanitary conditions is no use if a system of regular garbage collection and cleaning is not implemented. The desire for such a system is strongly linked with education.

## Employment

One of the social conditions mentioned above is safe occupational circumstances. Prevailing employment terms and conditions generally have an important influence on gender attitudes and reproductive health. This influence is best illustrated by comparing two hypothetical employment scenarios.

In the first scenario, a business starts up in a Scandinavian country where gender equality and good working terms and conditions are the norm. Under the terms of employment, a female employee is paid at the same rate as her male colleagues doing a similar job. She is allowed time off to attend her antenatal clinic and has the right to take a year off after delivering her baby and then to resume her employment.[22]

In the second scenario, a garment factory is owned by unscrupulous shareholders and is located in a very poor country where population pressure means that jobs are hard to obtain. Here the employees, nearly all women, are paid very little. Women are preferred to men because they are less expensive, more reliable, and less likely to revolt against the poor conditions. And the conditions are appalling. Employees are not allowed to stop work to go to the toilet except at the few designated breaks. Toilet facilities are basic and unhygienic; there are no showers or medical and recreation facilities. The employer posts no information on safety, medical, and reproductive health matters such as antenatal services and the risks and prevention of sexually transmitted infections, including HIV. The women are not only exploited as the cheapest source of labor but also are subject to abuse as well as unsafe working conditions. Such conditions could include improperly guarded or insulated equipment, exhaust fumes, dust, and so on. With a family to support, the employee's meager income is still too valuable for the employee to risk losing it by complaining. She has to accept abuse as "part of the job," and if she becomes pregnant, she is forced to continue as normal, is allowed no time off to attend an antenatal clinic, and will lose her job the day she goes into labor unless she returns the following day. The economic consequences for her and her family could be dire. In such circumstances, an overnight backstreet abortion becomes a viable option.

Unfortunately, the second scenario is all too real. The International Labour Organisation does have labor statistics (and is leading the fight to eliminate the use of child labor and to improve working conditions in poor countries, especially for women), but information is lacking on the effects on reproductive health of poor work terms and conditions—for example, the effects of pelvic inflammatory infection for which the female employees in the second work scenario are at risk because they are denied access to toilet facilities when needed. And pregnant employees have to forgo recommended antenatal care. They risk injury to themselves and their unborn child by performing tasks unsuitable for pregnant women. Employees who have recently delivered are denied the time or facility to attend to newborn babies. This situation is surely deserving of more attention and research.

Major international companies with production facilities in poor economies have responded to their customers' concerns about employees' working conditions and have made efforts to improve them. But there is a long way to go, especially in terms of dealing with medium-size and small businesses that are not subject to effective regulation or consumer pressure. The relationship between employment and reproductive health has evident links with education, community involvement, and public policy.

### Public Policy and Governance

Table 13.1 showed that countries with lower MMRs had better governance than those with higher rates, according to a governance effectiveness indicator. That indicator was one of six compiled by World Bank experts (Kaufmann and others 2003) for a study comparing 199 countries on the basis of several hundred variables drawn from 25 data sources. The other five indicators compiled by Bank staff are voice and accountability, political stability, regulatory capacity, rule of law, and control of corruption. The indicators have a mean of zero and a standard deviation of one, so that virtually all scores fall between –2.5 and +2.5; higher scores indicate better performance. In the MMR sample, few countries (the Bahamas, Singapore) had scores greater than one, and most were below the mean of zero. Table 13.2 presents the average scores by MMR group for each of the indicators. The table shows a consistent decline in performance as MMRs rise; the group with MMRs greater than 1,000 has an average score near or below one standard deviation below the mean for all of the indicators. Political instability stands out as the indicator with the lowest average for this group, and the highest average for the countries with low MMRs.

## Policy and Program Actions

The strong negative correlation between MMRs and per capita health expenditures suggests that more health spending is needed, but as the World Bank study on reaching the Millennium Development Goals (MDGs) in health reminds us, spending alone is not enough. The added health funding needs to be targeted to overcoming obstacles that reduce poor women's chances of accessing lifesaving interventions. Moreover, this funding has to be combined with improvements in government effectiveness and with motivation of individuals and communities to make use of these interventions. Sri Lanka and Malaysia demonstrate that sustained efforts to improve health system performance, increase women's education, and improve

**Table 13.2** Governance Indicators for Countries Grouped by MMR Level

| MMR level | Number of countries | Effective governance | Voice and accountability | Political stability | Regulatory quality | Rule of law | Control of corruption |
|---|---|---|---|---|---|---|---|
| 0–30 | 17 | 0.41 | .29 | .47 | .51 | .35 | .41 |
| 31–100 | 39 | −0.07 | −.24 | .04 | −.07 | −.12 | −.16 |
| 100–300 | 32 | −0.35 | −.23 | −.20 | −.27 | −.36 | −.40 |
| 301–1,000 | 41 | −0.37 | −.35 | −.37 | −.34 | −.38 | −.36 |
| Over 1,000 | 13 | −1.08 | −.86 | −1.13 | −1.07 | −1.06 | −.94 |

*Source:* Kaufmann and others 2003.

infrastructure, along with targeted investments and policy change to establish a cadre of trained midwives to ensure safe delivery and effective management of emergencies, can be successful (Pathmanathan and others 2003). Localities that have reduced maternal and neonatal mortality (Honduras and the Indian state of Kerala[23]) have proved that a combination of targeted investments in lifesaving interventions as well as social infrastructure can make a positive difference.

### Targeting the Poor

The marginal budgeting for bottlenecks (MBB) approach (described below) is based on the premise that increased public expenditure on health will have an even greater impact if targeted on key obstacles that prevent poor women from accessing lifesaving interventions. The first step in the MBB approach is identification of those obstacles (inside and outside the health system, beginning with individuals, households, and communities and including both health care and health financing as well as other sectors—education, transportation, water and sanitation, and nutrition). The next step is costing of interventions to address these obstacles, followed by tracking of expenditures and the performance of the interventions to ensure that the targeted spending is being used effectively and that the poor are benefiting.

Countries that have reduced mortality rates have done so through a combination of investments inside and outside the health system, including investments in improving the skills and deployment of midwives and other key staff, reducing financial obstacles to care, improving the quality of care and access to referral facilities, and mobilizing households and communities to ensure safe delivery and effective management of emergencies. Parallel investments in nutrition, malaria control, education, roads, and water and sanitation have also had a positive impact in situations in which low performance in those areas has undermined the reproductive health of poor women.

If use of interventions that are known to be effective could be increased from current levels to 99 percent, nearly four-fifths of the 529,000 maternal deaths that occur each year might be averted. The World Bank authors of *The Millennium Development Goals for Health: Rising to the Challenges* identified the changes that would be needed to ensure that these interventions are implemented, particularly in ways that benefit poor women (Wagstaff and Claeson 2004). A key question is whether additional government spending would help. One school of thought holds that added government spending is likely to have little effect because of corruption and the poor management of public services, but the authors of *The Millennium Development Goals for Health* take the view that added government spending could make a difference—provided it is combined with improvements in governance and is effectively targeted to the poor. They also call attention to the key role of households, both as consumers of health services and as producers of health outcomes, in ensuring that increases in delivery care will actually reduce maternal mortality and morbidity.

The study conducted by the World Bank authors employs a simulation modeling process to understand the possible impacts of increased government spending and improvements in government effectiveness as well as changes beyond the health sector (added economic growth, increased education, improved water supply) on achievement of the maternal mortality reduction target of the MDGs. The results are summarized in figure 13.1.

For each of the World Bank's Regions (the same regional breakdown as shown in the Demographic and Health Surveys tabulations), the figure

**Figure 13.1** *Possible Effects of Interventions on Achievement of the Maternal Mortality MDG in World Bank Regions*

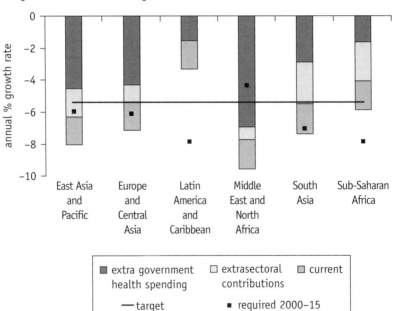

*Source:* Wagstaff and Claeson 2004.

shows the rate of decline in MMRs from 1990 to 2000 (labeled "current" with darker shading at top of bars) and the added decline that could occur (lighter shading at bottom of each bar) if an additional 2.5 percentage points were added to the annual growth of government health spending as a percentage of GDP, provided that countries achieve a level of effectiveness in governance that is one standard deviation above the mean of cross-national scores in the World Bank's Country Policy and Institutional Assessment (CPIA) data.[24] Figure 13.1 also shows (in the cross-hatched area in each bar) the potential contribution of extrasectoral contributions—added economic growth, better roads, quicker growth in female secondary schooling, and improved access to drinking water.

Finally, the figure shows the rates of decline between 1990 and 2015 that would be needed to meet the regional MDGs for reduced maternal mortality (the black line across the graph—5.75 percent annually) and the rates that would be needed between 2000 and 2015 for regions where declines were below the required level during the 1990–2000 period to reach the 2015 goal (the small black squares).

As the figure shows, only one region (the Middle East and North Africa) experienced declines in the MMR during the 1990s at a rate that would enable it to reach the 2015 MDG. All of the other regions need higher rates of increase during the 2000–15 period in order to catch up. In three regions (Europe and Central Asia, South Asia, and East Asia and Pacific) a combination of extrasectoral contributions and additional government health expenditures would bring the rate of decline up to the required level. In Sub-Saharan Africa, the projected impacts of the combination are just too weak, and in Latin America and the Caribbean, the levels of extrasectoral contributions are currently high enough that added change does not appear likely (though compared with other regions, MMR levels in the region are already low).

In making the case for increased health expenditures, the World Bank authors emphasize that they are talking not about across-the-board increases in expenditures but about targeted expenditures to increase the quality and accessibility of the key interventions needed to reduce the high maternal mortality experienced by poor women. *The Millennium Development Goals for Health* notes two promising approaches to such targeting. One of these is MBB, which targets added health expenditures to relieving bottlenecks in health system performance. The second is financing through social funds, which are targeted to improving the demand and capacities of poor localities and households where interventions need to occur.

MBB was developed by UNICEF, the World Bank, and WHO in conjunction with efforts to ensure that funds created by debt relief actually benefit the poor (Soucat and others 2004). It involves the formulation of national- or provincial-level medium-term expenditure plans that allocate newly available resources to achieve an MDG like reduced MMR. MBB uses proxy indicators from Demographic and Health Surveys and other data sources to identify five potential bottlenecks: gaps in physical accessibility, human resource bottlenecks, constraints related to supplies and logistics, demand and use constraints, and bottlenecks due to technical and organizational quality. In Mali, for example, the proportion of deliveries attended by trained staff was used as a performance measure and a costing and budgeting program was developed to reach an attended delivery "performance frontier." An epidemiological model was calculated to measure and then monitor the impact of increased expenditures on reaching this frontier.

Social funds (SFs) are agencies that finance small projects to benefit a country's poor and vulnerable groups. Projects are subject to specific eligibility criteria and are generated and managed by communities (Wagstaff and Claeson 2004). Evaluations of SFs in several countries have shown them to be effective mechanisms for channeling funding to poorer communities and for improving both the demand for and quality of health services. In Bolivia, for example, it was reported that medicines and essential drugs were more available in SF facilities. Moreover, by going beyond traditional approaches to investment in infrastructure, the SF increased use of services and contributed to a reduction in under-five mortality rates in SF communities (Newman and others 2002). An evaluation of the impact of social funds on health in four countries (Bolivia, Honduras, Nicaragua, and Zambia) found that SF health interventions had a positive impact on infrastructure quality and on the availability of medical equipment, furniture, and essential drugs. This impact, in turn, increased use of health facilities for critical services, including maternal and child health (Rawlings and others 2004).

## Other Government Policies

Other government policies that influence health outcomes include population growth policy, regional development, and social safety nets, as well as laws and regulations related to health facilities, inheritance, domestic violence, communicable diseases, abortion, employment and working conditions, child labor, prostitution, brewing and distilling, and pollution.

Other factors include the number and status of and conditions for health personnel: number and types of personnel undergoing training and continuing education, housing and other types of staff support, staff salaries, and regulation and control bodies such as the General Nursing Counsel. Mitigation of effects is related to donor policies such as restrictions on use of funds for contraceptives and abortion, rules related to generic drugs imposed by international drug companies, international declarations (for example, on child labor), and brain drain to rich countries with health personnel shortages.

# 14

## How to Win Friends and Influence People: Developing a Strategy for Change

The climate in which service providers and policy makers work is much more complex than it was 20 years ago. Hence, this last chapter in part 2 focuses on stakeholder analysis, an important tool for adaptation to changes in reproductive health policies and services and to health sector reforms in general. Such an analysis is crucial to attempts to influence various stakeholders.

### A Framework for Analyzing Stakeholders

Many actors influence country population and reproductive health policies and programs. The International Conference on Population and Development (ICPD) Program of Action, for example, was shaped by the influences of multiple players—governments, civil societies, international donor agencies, religious groups, and many others—who brought their very individual perspectives to bear. The same or similar groups will, to a greater or lesser extent, have an impact on whatever programs and services reproductive health advocates want to deliver in more localized settings.

How are the many stakeholders to be identified, and how can they be persuaded to come to an agreement that is beneficial to reproductive health when they represent differing opinions? For example, can the ministry of finance and the ministry of health, both of which want to introduce user fees for preventive care at the district level, ever agree with community consumer groups that say user fees will be detrimental to the health of poor women and children? How can common ground be found so that consensus can be reached?

Stakeholder analysis is a framework for identifying the various actors, assessing their importance, and developing strategies to gain their support (Walt and Gilson 1994). Brinkerhoff and Crosby (2002) define stakeholder analysis as a process that "assesses the nature of a policy's constituents, their interests, their expectations, the strength or intensity of their interest in the issue, and the resources they can bring to bear on the outcomes of a policy change." The framework below highlights the context, process, and stakeholders.

## Context

Context refers to systemic factors—political, economic, and social, both national and international—that may affect health policy. They include situational factors—more or less transient, impermanent, or idiosyncratic conditions such as wars and droughts—and structural factors—relatively unchanging features of a society such as the political system, type of economy and employment base, and demographics.[25] Context also includes cultural factors, such as ethnic minorities, religion, and linguistic differences, and international factors that lead to greater interdependence of and policy transfer among states (for example, internationally adopted goals such as the Millennium Development Goals).

## Process

Process refers to the way in which policies are initiated, formulated, negotiated, communicated, executed, and evaluated. Processes are commonly described in phases. In phase 1, problem identification and issue recognition, analysts explore how issues get onto the policy agenda and why some issues are never even discussed. In phase 2, policy formulation, analysts explore who should be involved, how the criteria for policy selection are determined, and how policies are developed, agreed on, and communicated to others. In phase 3, policy implementation, the most crucial phase (and often underestimated in policy making), resources are deployed to support scheduled actions and activities to make policy changes on a sustainable basis. In phase 4, policy evaluation, analysts identify what happens once a policy is implemented—how it is monitored, whether it has achieved the desired outcomes, whether it has had unintended consequences, and what further developments or changes are required.

In this description, the policy process appears linear. However, the process is rarely straightforward. It is iterative and is affected by the interests of a wide range of stakeholders.

### Stakeholders

Stakeholders are at the center of the policy analysis framework. They include individuals (the minister of health, for example), groups (advocacy groups), or individual organizations (such as a practitioners' association or a multilateral or bilateral organization). No organization is monolithic: the values and beliefs of the individuals working within an organization may differ.

A stakeholder analysis may be undertaken for many reasons. For example, it may be desirable to identify the policy position of various stakeholders involved in improving health system performance, particularly the position of those who are likely to have positive or negative influences on reproductive health outcomes. Identifying key policy issues is always useful for developing stakeholder strategies.

Stakeholder analysis helps reproductive health advocates understand, engage, and influence the stakeholders who shape policies. It helps them determine strategies for maintaining the support of current proponents and increasing the power and leadership of supporters. It also helps reproductive health advocates to convert opponents to supporters, weaken the power and leadership of opponents, and convert neutral stakeholders to active supporters. In short, stakeholder analysis helps reproductive health advocates be savvy about the politics of change.

Stakeholder analysis involves six steps: (1) identifying the issue, (2) determining the current phase of the policy process, (3) identifying stakeholders, (4) conducting stakeholder assessment (including self-assessment), (5) organizing and analyzing data (for example, positional mapping), and (6) determining strategies for action.

Identifying the Issue   Improving reproductive health is a multifaceted process and involves many policy issues that, in turn, may require many programmatic changes. Wider health sector reform is even more complex and will inevitably involve proposals with important implications for reproductive health and rights. Whatever the issue may be—cutting curative care at tertiary hospitals, transforming the health system from one that is centered on the ministry of health to one that is district–centered, cutting back on integrated management of childhood illness, introducing or eliminating user fees, or introducing provider payment incentives—reproductive health  advocates must be able to assess the risks and benefits for reproductive health and determine whether or not—and in what form—intervention is worthwhile.

The first step is to identify the policy issue on which efforts are to be focused. Several issues may need to be tackled, but one must be singled out to form the basis for resolving the others and, significantly, for bringing together disparate stakeholders.

Determining the Policy Process Phase   Identifying the current phase of the policy process, depicted in figure 14.1, is imperative to maximize the impact of a proposed intervention. An intervention is most likely to have the desired impact if it occurs at the policy formulation and legitimation phase or the implementation design and organizational structuring phase, although stakeholder interventions may also be effective at the constituency-building stage. Of course, multiple interventions at various stages could positively influence the process, depending on the desired result. For example, an input at the policy formulation stage is desirable to shape policy and at the implementation or constituency-building phase to maximize the support of the different stakeholders for the policy.

Identifying Stakeholders   The health policy process has both technical and sociopolitical dimensions; the interplay of political and technical issues is iterative rather than sequential. Both health reformers and champions of repro-

**Figure 14.1** Policy-Making Process

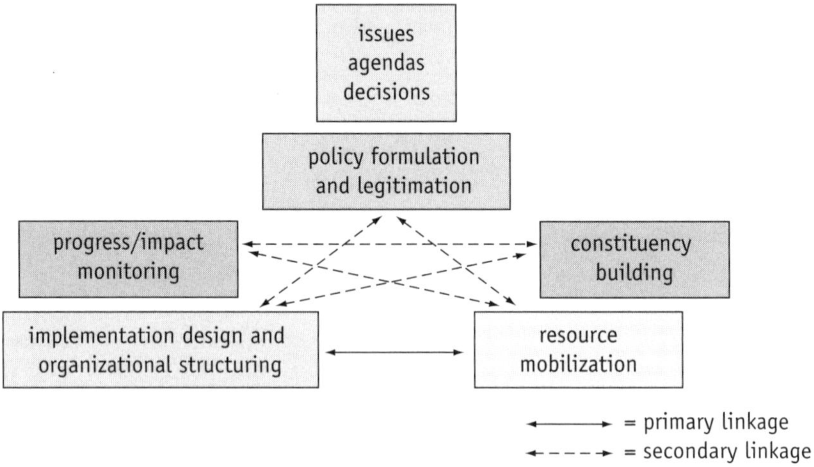

Source: USAID Partners for Health Reform Project.

ductive health tend to be technical experts who can make judgments about the "what," "why," and "how to" of health care. But those who influence whether initiatives are undertaken, financed, and supported in their implementation include both technical experts and a broader range of people. The latter may not be informed about or interested in the technical considerations that underlie a particular course of reform action, but they will voice opinions that could support or prevent, or otherwise affect, implementation.

Are stakeholders policy makers or policy advocates? The answer is either or both. And their positions may change as the policy-making process unfolds. So the next step in the stakeholder analysis is to identify the full range of stakeholders who will influence and be influenced by the policy in question and to understand how the policy will affect their interests and, therefore, how their views and behaviors are likely to affect the reform process (in this case, reform likely to affect reproductive health and rights).

Key stakeholders—who will have very different perspectives about the proposed policy issue—might include politicians, economists, donors and others who control financial resources, civil society, syndicates, unions and professional associations, individual providers, consumers (for example, women's health groups, individuals), the press, academicians, and so on. Their motivations vary:

- Politicians want to retain power and be reelected.
- Economists would like to see greater efficiency and are interested in the financial impact of the policy.
- Multilateral donors and charities are driven by goals and priorities set by their directors and managers and often determined by immediate needs.
- Bilateral donors in theory are accountable to their home country taxpayers but in practice are accountable to their government and are thus interested in favorable outcomes and the domestic policy response but are at times influenced by international politics.
- Professional organizations and labor unions do not want their posts to disappear and are interested in protecting not only their jobs but their working conditions and salaries.
- Civil society institutions, including religious groups, are likely to be most interested in rights and equity issues.
- Consumers desire quality services but often are uninformed about or disinterested in the proposed reform.
- The press wants a good story or an angle that presents the interests that direct them.

An understanding of what motivates different actors is crucial to knowing how to present options and proposals and, eventually, to influencing the policy-making process.

**Conducting Stakeholder Assessment**    Stakeholder assessment can employ a variety of techniques to identify and analyze stakeholder views: formal surveys, interviews with key informants, reviews of media reports, examination of key policy documents from affected organizations, Web site searches, organizational contacts and networking, and so on.

A key, and often neglected, component of stakeholder analysis is self-assessment. Self-assessment involves examining your own and your organization's power, interests, knowledge, skills, values, and position in relation to a given issue. The questions considered during a broader stakeholder analysis will still apply, but asking yourself some additional questions will help you maximize your strategic position. Box 14.1 presents a typical self-assessment exercise.

---

**Box 14.1** *Self-Assessment Exercise*

The ministry of health is considering a plan to introduce a fee for normal deliveries in dispensaries and tertiary care hospitals in order to mobilize extra funding for emergency deliveries that contribute greatly to maternal mortality in your country. What consequences would this decision have for reproductive health outcomes?

Given your current job, what is your position and that of your organization on the proposed introduction of this form of social insurance?

Using the following self-assessment questions, analyze your role as a stakeholder.

- What is your position?
- What are your interests?
- What is the extent of your power and influence and the basis of that power?
- What knowledge and skills can you bring to bear in making your case?
- What assistance might you need from allies and partners (and are they willing to provide it)?
- What flexibility do you have to negotiate alternatives? Are you in a position to offer practical alternatives?

*Source:* Authors.

Organizing and Analyzing Data    As stakeholder information is compiled, political mapping is helpful. Tools such as the "Policymaker" package developed at Harvard University are available online through the Management Sciences for Health Manager's Electronic Resource Center, as is the "Policy Toolkit for Strengthening Health Sector Reform" developed by the USAID's Partners for Health Reform (PHR) project. Figure 14.2 depicts a sample positional map from the PHR toolkit.

Once stakeholder data have been assembled, the next step is to consider questions such as the following:

- Who are the most important stakeholders in terms of power and leadership potential?

**Figure 14.2** *Sample Stakeholder Positional Map*

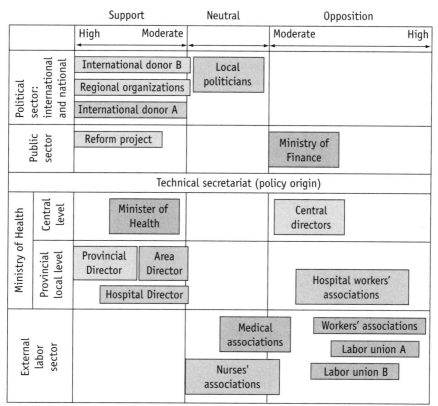

*Source:* USAID Partners for Health Reform Project.

- At what stage and in what ways are they involved in the decision-making process?
- What do the stakeholders know about the policy?
- What positions have they taken on the policy?
- What do they perceive to be the advantages and disadvantages of the policy in relation to their own interests?
- Do they have any other interests (secondary or peripheral) that might influence their behavior?
- Which stakeholders have or might form alliances with reproductive health advocates?
- Which stakeholders might ally against reproductive health advocates?

All stakeholders are important. Those who today are less influential may be leaders tomorrow, and groups of stakeholders may form alliances to promote their common views.

On the basis of stakeholder analysis, including self-assessment, reproductive health advocates can determine their own and allies' capacity to influence each stakeholder's position and use this knowledge to develop a framework for managing the information collected about the various actors.

In the hypothetical case of a proposal to introduce user fees (box 14.1), the next step would be to identify other stakeholders with an interest in this issue. The following stakeholders are likely to be involved: ministry of health officials, private providers, donors, the World Bank, nurses and doctors' associations, local and district-level politicians, consumers, NGOs, and district health officers. Having identified these stakeholders, the next step is to assess the degree to which they can or are likely to influence policy. The result might look something like that depicted in table 14.1.

These stakeholders probably represent a wide range of views on the issue, so it is useful to map their likely position, as depicted in table 14.2.

**Table 14.1** *Stakeholders' Levels of Power*

| High | Medium | Low |
|------|--------|-----|
| Ministry of Health | NGOs | Consumers |
| Doctors' associations | Donors | Private providers |
| World Bank | District health officials | Nurses' associations |
| | Local and district-level politicians | |

*Source:* Authors.

**Table 14.2** *Stakeholders' Positions*

| Support | Neutral | Opposition |
|---|---|---|
| Donors | Ministry of Health | Local and district-level politicians |
| District health officials | Nurses' associations | Consumers |
| Doctors' associations | Private providers | |

*Source:* Authors.

Some of the stakeholders may be well informed, but others less so. To be able to influence their views, it is important to assess the extent of their knowledge, as shown in table 14.3.

With this assessment, it is possible to consider which alliances are likely to be forged (table 14.4).

Determining Strategies for Action   Armed with the stakeholder analysis, especially the information displayed in the mapping exercise, reproductive health advocates can develop communications, advocacy, alliance building, and negotiating strategies. These strategies should be designed to engage as many stakeholders as possible in actions to correct distortions and implementation problems that could have adverse effects on reproductive health and rights. The emergent strategies could, for example, include facilitating

**Table 14.3** *Stakeholders' Knowledge*

| High | Medium | Low |
|---|---|---|
| District health officials | NGOs | Consumers |
| World Bank | Donors | Private providers |
| | Doctors' associations | Local and district-level politicians |
| | Nurses' associations | Ministry of Health |

*Source:* Authors.

**Table 14.4** *Stakeholders' Alliances*

| Support | Opposition |
|---|---|
| Ministry of Health | NGOs |
| District health officials | Consumers |
| Doctors' associations | Local and district-level politicians |

*Source:* Authors.

an informed and open consensus-building process, making strategic changes in personnel or the implementation process, and creating or strengthening selected alliances.

## Consumers as Stakeholders

The rights-based approach that characterized the ICPD was a direct result of the involvement of civil society. Since the ICPD, consumer interest groups have had an increasing voice in bringing about changes in reproductive health policies and practices. Consumers can therefore be powerful allies for reproductive health advocates. Hence, the obstacles to and opportunities for community participation in reproductive health and health sector reform should be fully considered when formulating strategies for action. From a strategic perspective, consumers are the users and beneficiaries of reproductive health services and, ultimately, are the most important stakeholders. Ensuring representative and effective community involvement is therefore desirable.

Reproductive health advocates should be aware of the difficulties and risks of consumer participation. Typically, the most significant problem is finding the right balance of interested groups. Organizations represent differing numbers of persons as well as different interests. Some will be professional groups (small but powerful) that may be well informed but have self-interests as well as consumer interests to consider, and they may have a tendency to crowd out less well-informed consumer voices. Collaboration of government interest groups could hamper the participation of poorer segments of the population. Consumer groups are often poorly informed and, in some settings, their constituents may be illiterate and need access to alternative types of educational materials. The poor and vulnerable may be badly organized, if they are organized at all; they may have little tradition of participation in advocacy efforts or negotiations and little time to spare for these activities.

Individuals will represent these various interest groups. Some of them may be highly articulate, some outspoken, others retiring, some influential, and others less so. Thus, the interaction of personalities is yet another factor that must be taken into account in deciding how to disseminate ideas, information, and proposals. Ensuring the inclusion of the right people becomes an art as well as a science, especially if some groups are underrepresented or not represented at all. Reproductive health advocates should ask the questions: who are the poor, and who represents them?

Despite the complexities of involving consumers in policy formulation and implementation, doing so will increase the likelihood that services will be used and equitably distributed and, therefore, will strengthen the policy's legitimacy.

## Benefits and Costs of Increased Stakeholder Participation

Stakeholder analysis can be a valuable tool if well designed and properly implemented. However, it can be complex and time consuming. So, before proceeding, reproductive health advocates should consider the following:

- Will increased stakeholder participation improve the technical content of the policy, enhance the legitimacy of the policy, and increase ownership of the policy?
- Is support from the stakeholder(s) required to adequately design or implement the policy? How much support will be needed? What kind of support will be required?
- Will including the stakeholder(s) in the formulation phase dilute the policy's objectives or compromise the intended impacts?
- Conversely, to what extent would exclusion of one or more groups weaken the policy formulation and implementation processes and the desired outcomes?
- Can the organization(s) managing the participation process meet the stakeholders' expectations (for participation and outcomes)? What level of participation will be required to satisfy these expectations?
- At which stage in the policy process is the stakeholders' participation most helpful or necessary (formulation or implementation or both)?
- What are the actual or potential conflicts among the stakeholders' views and expectations and the demands of other stakeholders?
- How much additional time will be required to incorporate each of the stakeholders into the policy process? Are there fixed deadlines and timetables that needed to be considered?
- Are the benefits of including the stakeholder likely to outweigh the costs?

# PART III
## *From Victims of Reform to Drivers of Reform*

# 15

## Shotgun Wedding: Reproductive Health and Health Sector Reform

Chapter 1 described a large health system failure that has led to many global health initiatives and a health sector reform agenda. This chapter and the two that follow examine what is typically meant by health sector reform and how it both creates an opportunity for the reproductive health agenda as well as poses a threat.

### The Health Reform Agenda

Health sector reform conjures dramatically different images in the minds of donors and policy makers. Participants in the World Bank Institute's Reproductive Health and Health Sector Reform program[26] find reform difficult to define. Some focus on cost recovery, while others mention payment mechanisms or decentralization. More interesting and revealing than the lack of consensus, is the majority of the participants' view that reform is bad for the International Conference on Population and Development (ICPD) agenda. Yet the only way that agenda, at least the part that deals with provision of services and choices, can be achieved is if health systems are dramatically improved. Health sector reforms, defined generically, can be tools for strengthening health systems (Krasovec and Shaw 2000).

Health sector reform has been researched, evaluated, vilified, praised, defined, and reviewed to death over the last 20 years.[27] Regardless of where we stand on specific reforms or the health sector reform agenda, failure to understand these reforms or to engage in them is likely to undermine reproductive health objectives.

Consider popular reforms such as decentralization, which focuses on the overall organization and management of health service delivery in the public sector. Decentralization is typically driven by political issues outside the health sector, but it can have a profound impact, positive or negative, on health systems and outcomes. A decentralization process that empowers informed local decision making and that allows women and the poor to fully participate in the accountability mechanism of service delivery is likely to have a positive impact on reproductive health. On the other hand, a decentralization process can lead to the capture of decision-making and accountability mechanisms by local elites who are hostile to reproductive health concerns (World Bank 2003b).

The technical dimensions of reforms are equally important. If decentralization of health services did not take into account functions that cut across more than one level of care, such as referral, reproductive health outcomes could deteriorate, even if accountability issues are well addressed. Actors must be identified and functions mapped to ensure that the different levels of the system are reinforced and provide all the critical functions. Failure to address these functions at the design stage and to implement monitoring mechanisms to ensure they are covered will produce negative outcomes for health, including reproductive health.

The main message for the reproductive health community is not to view reform as negative but to participate in the design and implementation of reform of health systems that are failing poor people, especially poor women. In fact, the failures of the health system should propel the reform agenda. The reproductive health community can use its knowledge of the technical dimensions of reform to be the driver of reform instead of the victim.

## What Is Health Sector Reform?

The 1990s brought a rethinking of how governments and donor agencies approach health. A combination of factors—rising costs, scarcity of resources, lack of impact of health spending on health status, growing health problems (including a resurgence of old infections and an emergence of new ones), and anticipated shifts in burden of disease as populations age and adopt new lifestyles—revealed major fault lines in traditional modes of financing and organizing public sector involvement in health. Reforms are being undertaken for a variety of reasons:

- *Improving health, even in resource-poor settings:* Despite advances in disease control and improvements in life expectancy, the health status of poor populations remains precarious. Infections such as malaria and tuberculosis inflict a serious disease burden. The HIV/AIDS epidemic is spreading rapidly. The gap between rich and poor countries has widened for health indicators such as maternal mortality. One of the main goals of reforms is to lay the groundwork for narrowing this gap.

- *Mobilizing resources to improve health and ensuring that these resources are allocated efficiently and used effectively:* Resources for health are very limited in poor countries. Existing resources need to be used more effectively; new ones need to be mobilized through affordable, equitable, and efficient risk pooling (complemented by appropriate user charges) and by maintaining effective expenditure controls in both the public and private sectors. Reform efforts seek to improve both the technical and allocative efficiency of resource use.

- *Ensuring that subsidies benefit poor and vulnerable groups:* Public subsidies are often skewed toward curative services in major cities, benefiting middle- and upper-income classes more than the poor in both urban or rural areas. One goal of reform is to ensure that subsidies benefit poor and vulnerable groups and that those who can pay for services do so through cost recovery and risk sharing initiatives.

- *Improving the quality and client focus of public and private health services:* The poor quality of publicly provided health services has often led consumers to pay for substandard care in the private sector. More resources are needed to improve quality, but much can also be done through better management and improved accountability.

## What Does "Reform" Mean?

Berman (1995) has defined health reform as "sustained, purposeful change to improve the efficiency, equity and effectiveness of the health sector." At the country level, reform initiatives to address these goals include

- decentralizing budgeting and management of service delivery (local managers rather than ministry officials make staffing and spending decisions);

- separating financing from provision of services, thereby opening the way for government to contract with private providers for service delivery and to hold them accountable for performance;

- new financing and payment schemes, including service fees and social and private insurance systems;
- devolving ownership and management of tertiary care facilities to private nonprofit or commercial organizations and allowing community oversight through local health boards and other mechanisms;
- shifting donor financing from inputs/projects to results-oriented, policy-based sectoral program support; and
- reorganizing ministries of health and redefining roles of central units to shift them from management of service delivery to standard setting, advocacy, and evaluation.

These actions can improve efficiency, effectiveness, and equity in service delivery, but they inevitably involve trade-offs. As countries implement reforms, they need to ensure that health systems maintain the quality and accessibility of reproductive health care. They also need to strengthen human resources and management capacity at all system levels.

Figure 15.1 maps health system functions and identifies actors. As the figure indicates, consumers pay for health services through taxes, insurance premiums, and out-of-pocket payments. Consumers also produce health. As we learned in chapter 6, healthy behaviors are a key determinant of health outcomes.

Consumer payments in taxes and insurance premiums are channeled through health financing institutions. These institutions include public and private insurance organizations as well as national and subnational government ministries and agencies that pay for health care. In some countries,

**Figure 15.1** Health System Functions, Actors, and Payment Mechanisms

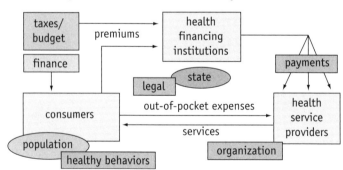

*Source:* Authors.

private enterprises collect and disburse payments for health care on behalf of their employees.

As will be described in chapter 17, payment for health care can take several forms: government budget, fees for services, and contracts between providers and insurance organizations (for example, capitation agreements through which a provider agrees to make a specific package of services available to a specific population for a specific period for an agreed price). The form of payment is important, because it affects provider motivation and performance. It also affects consumer behavior. Shifts in the way payments are made can change incentives such that service performance and health outcomes improve.

The ways in which providers are organized and manage services is another important dimension of health system performance. In some health systems, providers are public sector employees whose salaries are covered by government budgets. In other health systems, providers are private sector employees who may be paid by insurance organizations or directly by consumers through service fees or other payment schemes, such as capitation. Organization changes—for example, shifting the control and management of public services from the national to the local level or from the public to the private sector—are another type of reform and will be described in chapter 16.

In addition to financier and provider of health services, the state may also play an important regulatory role in health systems by setting standards for service provision, regulating medicines, and accrediting health providers. The state may delegate some of these functions to nongovernmental organizations (NGOs)—for example, to professional associations.

Reform, as the role of the state reminds us, is an intensely political process, because it affects the interests of consumers as well as providers, and any change in incentives involves trade-offs in which there will be both winners and losers. One of our concerns is that changes affecting reproductive health information and services will not result in poor women and children becoming losers in the reform process.

## Assessing the Impact of Reforms on Reproductive Health

How can the champions of reproductive health ensure that reforms work for rather than undermine reproductive health? They need to recognize that health reform is not a "black box" but a series of measures that countries implement to improve the performance of their health systems. The first step in assessing the impact of country-level reforms on reproductive health is to understand the problems that the reforms are attempting to address and how reformers expect the changes they promote to improve health system performance.

One entry point into this process is to examine how reformers measure success. Figure 15.2 depicts a framework employed by reformers to diagnose health system ills and assess the impact of reforms on both system performance and health outcomes. In the framework, the health system functions described above (financing, payment mechanisms, organization, and regulation) are considered health reform "levers" or mechanisms through which health policy changes could improve performance problems. The framework focuses on three sets of changes that might result from applying these levers: changes in system inputs, changes in system process, and changes in outcomes. In the framework, the impact of these changes is assessed in terms of success criteria, including access to and quality of services, equity and efficiency of service delivery, and sustainability and accountability. Figure 15.2 depicts a few health outcomes, improvements in which are the ultimate goal of health system reform. This framework can help the reproductive health community track the impact of reforms on reproductive health.

**Figure 15.2** *Framework for Diagnosing Health System Ills and Assessing the Impact of Reforms*

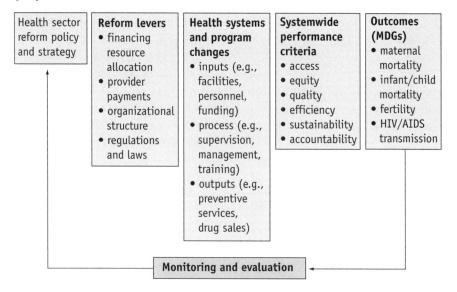

*Source:* LSMS 2000 (Instituto Cuánto 2000).

Table 15.1 presents the reform process in terms of the poor reproductive health outcomes that countries may be experiencing and some of the underlying flaws in the health system that may be contributing to these outcomes. Country case examples are cited to illustrate ways in which reproductive health risks have been addressed.

## Organizational Changes

Uganda illustrates one of the most common types of organizational change—decentralization—and the risks associated with this type of restructuring.[28] Decentralization of Uganda's public health services has taken place within the framework of the overall decentralization of the public sector. Most health facilities have been transferred to district governments; the Ministry of Health retains functions such as policy formulation, regulation, standard setting, and technical support to the districts. Recurrent and capital budgets have been transferred to districts, and different types of grant programs have been established to address special health needs.

Adequate financing of priority maternal and neonatal services across districts in Uganda proved to be an issue in the decentralization process. Because decentralization and district-level resource allocation involved all sectors and not just health, and because district managers perceived that health was relatively well funded, they tended to spend their funds on activities other than health. The Ministry of Health responded by establishing district-level grants to ensure that priority programs were adequately funded. Donor funding for several of the programs—for example, family planning, HIV/AIDS, and safe motherhood—supplemented these grants. The grants helped Uganda maintain the level of reproductive health care that had been established earlier and contributed to the country's effective mobilization to address its HIV/AIDS epidemic (Mirembe, Ssengooba, and Lubanga 1998).

Another common issue in decentralization is the capacity of local health managers to address reproductive health issues. When administrative and financial management of reproductive health programs shifts from the Ministry of Health to local managers, these managers will need technical support and guidance. When reformers in Zambia did away with the central maternal and child health unit, some district managers had no skills to manage reproductive health programs. Zambia corrected this problem by developing a national reproductive health strategy and setting up a system to provide technical support and guidance on reproductive health matters for district managers.[29]

*Table 15.1* *Assessing Health Reform Impacts on Reproductive Health*

| | | | | |
|---|---|---|---|---|
| **Poor outcomes** | High maternal mortality and morbidity<br>High prevalence of reproductive tract infections<br>High rates of unplanned/unwanted fertility | | | |
| **Flaws in health system** | Inequitable access to services and information<br>Scarcity of resources for health/reproductive health<br>Public spending that does not benefit the poor<br>Poor-quality services that do not address consumer needs<br>Waste and inefficiency in resource use | | | |
| **Type of reform and example** | **Organization:** Decentralized management of system | **Financing:** User fees | **Payments and incentives:** Contracts for private providers | **Laws and regulations:** New service delivery norms |
| **How reform is expected to improve the health system** | The system will become more responsive to local needs: more local ownership and accountability | Getting nonpoor to pay for services will increase resources for the poor | Salaried public sector workers often not motivated; contracting may improve performance | Norms can ensure that national policies are implemented in decentralized systems |
| **Potential risks for reproductive health** | Local managers may not view reproductive health as a priority and thus fail to fund key services | Poor women may be denied services for lack of enough money | Contracts may bias incentive schemes in favor of the nonpoor | Local managers may not adhere to norms or spend funds allocated to reproductive health |
| **How risks could be mitigated** | Reproductive health advocacy to ensure funding though district-level block grants for reproductive health (Uganda) | Assess the equity impact of financing schemes; risk pooling rather than user fees (Niger) | Incentives and more flexible payment schemes (Bolivia's maternal health program) | Advocacy and oversight of laws, regulations, and funding by women's health groups (Brazil) |

## Financing

Niger's experience with alternative financing models illustrates the importance of assessing the impact of alternative approaches on equity. Many countries have experimented with user fees to recover a portion of the costs of health services and medicines. Many concerns have been voiced about the adverse impact of these fees on poor people's access to health care.[30] To address such concerns, Niger experimented with two alternative cost recovery methods: a fee-for-service model and a type of social financing or risk sharing based on a combination of annual prepayments and fees. Niger hoped that cost recovery in the rural health system would improve the quality and accessibility of services for poor women and children. An analysis of the equity impact of the alternatives showed that the social financing approach had a more positive impact than the fee-for-service approach and had greater prospects for sustainability.[31]

## New Payment and Incentive Schemes

Bolivia's health strategy decentralized management of health interventions and sought to improve the amount and effectiveness of public spending by creating a payment scheme (Seguro Nacional de Maternidad y Niñez or SNMN) aimed at reducing economic barriers for poor women and children by eliminating copayments for key maternal and child health interventions. SNMN guaranteed free treatment and medicines in participating health facilities to treat many conditions of women and of children under five. These institutions included Ministry of Health facilities at all levels of the service delivery system, some social security hospitals, and a small number of private NGOs. Municipal governments reimbursed facilities for drugs, supplies, hospitalization, and lab exams for covered services. Rates are based on the average costs of treating the conditions using Ministry of Health protocols and are subject to approval by local health directorates.

Use of covered services increased after implementation of SNMN, but noncoverage of supply, labor, and capital costs posed a serious disincentive to providers outside the Ministry of Health system. Although Ministry of Health facilities could recover these costs through other government resource allocation channels, NGOs had to find ways to pay for them elsewhere and without charging for services in order to be reimbursed under SNMN. Social security facilities faced similar problems and reacted by rationing care for SNMN patients and erecting artificial barriers to clients seeking care under SNMN. In reality, part of the cost was being passed on to consumers, particularly through payments for medications.

An evaluation of SNMN by the Partners for Health Reform recommended several solutions, including incentives for providers who meet quality and client satisfaction standards, more flexible payment schemes for private providers, and user charges for people who are able to pay.[32]

### Laws and Regulations

Brazil's experience with health reform illustrates the importance of attention to the legal and regulatory frameworks in order to protect reproductive health and rights during the reform process. Brazil's reforms began during the 1980s with the dismantling of centralized national health finance/provision schemes and the devolution of facilities and personnel to states and municipalities. Free services for all citizens were to be financed through a revenue-sharing scheme under the new Unified Health System, which included a program of reproductive and child health services. Implementation of the program was undermined by the political and economic turmoil of the late 1980s.

During the early 1990s, Brazilian women's health advocates played a major role in promoting reproductive health and rights issues both at home and in international forums such as the ICPD and the Fourth World Conference on Women. Political action and advocacy for issues such as family planning and abortion legislation and norms, as well as for adequate funding and actual use of funds by local health officials, helped ensure that reproductive health was integrated into municipal-level primary health services once political and economic stability returned in the mid-1990s. In Brazil, the major principles underlying health reform—universal access, comprehensive care, equity, decentralization, and social accountability—were made to work for rather than against reproductive health and rights by highly effective community advocates working at various levels of the health system.[33]

## Making Reform Work for Reproductive Health

To ensure that the potential of health reforms to improve reproductive health is realized, the champions of reproductive health and rights need to understand the reform process, assess the risks to reproductive health associated with reforms, and act strategically to mitigate those risks. Rather than view reform as a threat, reproductive health advocates need to engage in the reform process through a variety of mechanisms:

- *Establishing clear program goals and agreed, measurable indicators of progress toward these goals:* One of the main shifts under reform is from program inputs to program results. Consequently, key stakeholders (community and women's groups as well as those responsible for reproductive health care) need to be involved in the goal-setting and indicator selection process. They also need to be involved in establishing the annual sectorwide operational and expenditure plans that include the program elements for which they can provide technical support and oversight. The mechanisms for this involvement need to be built into the program management structure at an early stage.
- *Involving the user community in program design, management, and oversight:* Another hallmark of both health reform and the reproductive health agenda is greater focus on the needs/demand of users of health services in the design and management of those services. In addition to participatory "log frame" processes, many other quantitative and qualitative methodologies (for example, focus groups, service delivery surveys, and household demand surveys) can be used to assess and reconcile the interests of stakeholders in the reform process. Although attribution of outcomes to specific reform initiatives is not easy, careful selection of indicators will help those concerned about reproductive health and rights monitor the impact of changes on desired outcomes.[34]
- *Ensuring adequate financial and technical support for priority program areas:* In prereform settings, maternal and child health/family planning units (MCH/FP) typically prepare subsectoral plans and budgets for items such as salaries, equipment, supplies, facilities, training, and external technical experts. Under reform, most of the responsibility for planning and budgeting passes to regional/local managers, sectorwide planning units, or both. At this level, managers typically do not (indeed cannot) allocate expenditures such as salaries and facilities to functional categories like MCH/FP. Units that formerly looked out for the interests of these subsectors by controlling budget lines will still need to assure themselves and donors that allocations to reproductive health are adequate. In the face of competition for scarce resources, they need to demonstrate that such services are in demand and needed and that the services are cost effective (that is, they are getting good results for monies spent). They

also have to ensure that key inputs such as contraceptives and other reproductive health drugs, specialized training, behavior change communications, and technical expertise are available to support effective service delivery.

- *Taking part in change management to ensure an effective transition process:* Implementation of reforms and introduction of integrated reproductive health services delivery involve many changes in the organization and management of health systems. Many countries have established change management units to bring in experts to help assess and strengthen organizational capacity building, personnel systems, and financial management. Reproductive health interests need to be represented in such units.

- *Attending to reproductive health in establishing donor codes/compacts to ensure appropriate donor behaviors:* Reformers are concerned that donors can undermine a reform effort by refusing to play by the new rules or by reverting to old modes of assistance that work against key elements of the reform agenda (for example, vertical programs that do not fit in with agreed sectoral goals or that distort agreed operational and expenditure programs). Reformers could view donor funding and technical support for reproductive health as a threat if reproductive health managers have not coordinated their efforts with those of the broader reform program. Some may believe that it is easier to get results by "going it alone," but a coordinated approach is likely to lead to better and more sustainable interventions, particularly in areas such as maternal health care and STD prevention, which depend on referral and other supporting services.

Health reform and efforts to improve and expand reproductive health services can and should be, but are not guaranteed to be, mutually reinforcing. Both require changes in the way of doing business. Champions of reproductive health cannot leave design and implementation of reforms to health economists. They must be "at the table" when reforms are being discussed. They need to employ the language and analytical tools of the reform movement to track the ways in which specific reform measures are affecting reproductive health outcomes. Moreover, they must demonstrate to reformers that correcting distortions when they arise will help countries achieve the shared goals of mobilizing resources, more cost-effectively and equitably using resources, and improving reproductive health.

# 16

*Slipping through the Cracks: Organizational Reform and Reproductive Health*

Governments are undertaking reforms in the organization and management of health services for a variety of reasons. Evaluations of health system performance have revealed many problems, including waste and inefficiency resulting from the poor management of service delivery, lack of responsiveness to client needs and poor client orientation in service delivery, and inequities in access to services.

For many people organizational reform connotes decentralization, as noted in chapter 10. Yet organizational reform spans a broader range of undertakings, including changes in the roles of government and the private sector in health system functions (financing, management of inputs, provision, norms, and regulations) and changes in responsibilities and reporting relationships among levels of government—national, state/province, local—and between government and the private sector. This chapter examines organization changes, their risks and benefits, and their potential effects on reproductive health (using a case study from the Philippines). In addition, it identifies some lessons from a variety of experiences to help ensure that organizational reforms work for rather than undermine reproductive health.

Health systems around the world differ with respect to the roles of government and the private sector in the health system functions depicted in figure 15.1. In some countries the government mobilizes and pools resources and also pays providers through taxes, government budget mechanisms, and social insurance. In other countries private insurance companies collect premiums and pay providers. In many cases, we find a mix of public and private involvement in these roles, usually as a result of organizational reforms.

What kinds of change do organizational reforms bring about? As the next chapter will explain, one of the main ways in which countries whose government has played the lead role in health seek to improve the performance of their health systems is by splitting the financing and provision functions. In countries where government will continue to play the lead role in financing and provision, improved performance may be sought by shifting authority for staff deployment and expenditure allocation decisions to lower levels of government.

Most often, organizational reform involves a variety of changes, for example, decentralization and a concomitant increase in the role of the private sector through contracts and other arrangements. Chapter 10 presented one example of organizational change: integration of "vertical" health programs—programs freestanding with respect to financing, input management, and provision—into a package of services or benefits.

## Decentralization

Decentralization can take three forms. The first and mildest form is *deconcentration*, or the transfer of authority and responsibility from the central to the field offices of an agency. The second form, *devolution*, is the transfer of authority and responsibility from central government to lower levels of government through statutory or constitutional measures. Devolution in the health sector usually occurs when decentralization in the country is governmentwide, so that the locus of control over many public sector functions (education, roads, and communications, as well as health) shifts to a lower level of government. The third form of decentralization is *delegation*, or the transfer of authority and responsibility from central agencies to organizations outside their direct control. Contracting service delivery to private providers is a form of delegation. Figure 16.1 illustrates some of the ways government and health ministry decentralization can occur.

Like other reforms, decentralization is not a magic bullet. Reformers need to examine the pros and cons of decentralization for each health system function and identify potentially adverse effects on key health system goals: equity, quality, efficiency, financial sustainability, and responsiveness to consumers.

**Figure 16.1** *Forms of Decentralization for Government and Health Ministries*

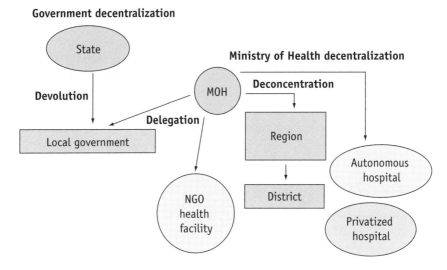

*Source:* Leighton and others 2002.

Consider the benefits and drawbacks of shifting control of resource allocations to subnational units. This change may correct some of the imbalances associated with overly centralized control. However, as the experience of India has shown, the net effect may be to maintain, and possibly worsen, resource inequities if richer localities can mobilize more of their own resources than poor localities.

Deconcentration may give local managers more control over input management, such as purchase of medicines, maintenance of facilities and equipment, hiring and deployment of staff, and contracting with vendors. But their ability to implement these decisions will depend on whether they have access to financial resources or retain revenue generated by fees, if they collect them, rather than return funds to the national treasury. In many instances, broader regulations may restrict the capacity of local managers to exercise the decision-making authority that reforms have granted them.

Decentralization in the health sector may occur as part of broader initiatives that give greater autonomy to local governments through devolution. The degree to which this shift occurs will depend on the political structure of the country in question. Local autonomy may already exist to some degree in large countries (India, Brazil, and Nigeria, for example) with a federal government, national and state/provincial governments, and district/municipal governments. When the power of the purse has been devolved to local governments, local health authorities will compete for resources with other branches of local government—education, roads, the police, parks and recreation, and so on.

Decentralization is an intensely political process. The form it takes, as well as the associated risks and benefits, including those for reproductive health, will depend on the political system in which it is undertaken. No single formula can adequately capture the range of circumstances and issues associated with decentralization. For that we must look to countries' experience with it.

### *Devolution—The Philippines Experience*

The Philippines decided to devolve many government functions to local governments. Although resisted by the Department of Health (DOH), responsibility for delivery, management, and financing of health services was shifted to the district level. Overall funding was allocated to district governments using a formula based on population and land area, and these governments were given wide discretion to allocate funds to health or other uses. Health represented 65 percent the total cost of devolved national government functions (Lakshminarayanan 2003).

In less than two years, 95 percent of facilities, 60 percent of personnel, and 45 percent of budget were transferred from the DOH to 1,600 local government units. The transition was not smooth. Technical and referral links between rural health units at the municipal level and primary/secondary facilities at district and province levels were disrupted, and reproductive health skills eroded as technical support weakened. After the shift to the local level, health worker salaries fell as much as 40 percent lower than those in the private sector before devolution.

Health system devolution in the Philippines had five unintended consequences for the quality and financing of reproductive health services. First, funding for curative care crowded out preventive care. Second, funding and coverage mechanisms to remove financial barriers for the poor disappeared. Third, many municipalities experienced a chronic lack of equipment and drugs. Fourth, cuts in travel allowances reduced supervision of rural and municipality-based midwives. Fifth, local governments were more conservative about reproductive health issues, and women were underrepresented in priority setting.

Lakshminarayanan (2003) has argued that these negative effects were not a direct result of devolution per se but that they resulted from the failure of policy makers and implementers to prepare adequately for devolution. Her view is that the national government should have defined a core package of reproductive health services to be made universally available and accessible. The absence of such a package allowed local officials to ignore reproductive health services if political or religious pressures made it convenient to do so. Similar problems arising from lack of support for reproductive health by local leaders were reported in a review of the impact of the devolution process in Senegal (Wilson 2000).

To have prevented or mitigated the above-noted negative effects, the Philippines DOH could have employed cost-sharing arrangements, provided better training and technical assistance mechanisms, implemented more effective regulatory mechanisms such as accreditation, better designed health benefit products under the national health insurance program, and addressed weak capacity in the health system. In addition, the department could have played a more constructive role in establishing new directions in reproductive health care by encouraging cooperation among localities and promoting better coordination between its own facilities and devolved local operations.

Comprehensive health care agreements between the Department of Health and local governments turned out to be ineffective in influencing the priorities of local government units because of a lack of incentives and sanctions, supporting policies to protect the poor, and training on new roles and functions. Moreover, the allocation formula did not consider local cost needs, capacities, and revenue-generating capacity.

The Philippines experience demonstrates that organization change requires careful planning and a lot of technical support and capacity building, including a specific focus on reproductive health issues, if reproductive health services are to improve.

### Delegation

Even when society agrees that the public sector should be responsible for the health of its citizens, the government may contract with NGOs and the private commercial sector to carry out health system functions, including financing, input management, and provision. Countries may decide to let market forces shape functions but can counteract market failures through regulation, standards, and targeted subsidies.

Loevinsohn and Harding (2005) have reviewed the experiences of many countries in which government contracted with nonstate entities, including NGOs, to improve the quality of health care delivery. They argue that contracting offers potential benefits that include focusing on results; overcoming the absorptive capacity problems that often plague governments; providing greater flexibility and efficiency as a result of competition; and enabling governments to attend to oversight, regulation, and public health functions. At the same time, Loevinsohn and Harding note contracting's possible pitfalls, including problems of scaling up, managing and sustaining contracting relationships, greater transaction costs, and inequality of access to care. Table 16.1 summarizes Loevinsohn and Harding's findings on contracting experiences in several countries.

Loevinsohn and Harding report that in 6 of 10 studies contracted services were more effective than the government on the basis of criteria such as quality of care, coverage, and cost effectiveness. They also reported findings for Cambodia, where the Ministry of Health tried two approaches to contacting: (1) contracting with NGOs to manage district-level health care delivery (contracting out) and (2) contracting with NGOs to assist district managers in delivery of a service package (contracting in). Because some districts continued to use the old model of government management and delivery, Loevinsohn and Harding were able to compare results of all three approaches. Their evaluation showed that contracting out led to better and more equal coverage for a range of maternal and child health services, including immunizations, antenatal care, modern birth spacing, and delivery in a facility.

## Decision Space

Researchers who study decentralization and its effect on health system performance have employed the concept of "decision space" to determine the degree to which local managers have decision-making authority for various health system functions. Table 16.2 illustrates the application of this concept in four countries.

Looking at decentralization in this way enables those concerned about the impact of reforms to track both the potential benefits and the risks of changes, for example:

- Local managers can be more aware of local health needs and financial requirements and therefore can make more efficient management decisions than distant bureaucrats, but they may also be subject to

**Table 16.1** Contracting Experiences

| Location and type of services (ref) | Type of contract and intervention | Scale and cost | Evaluation methodology | Main results | Subsequent history |
|---|---|---|---|---|---|
| 1. Cambodia Rural PHC and district hospital services | SDC compared to MC and CC (i.e., government provision of services) | 1.5 million Cost per head per year SDC = $4.50 MC = $2.82 CC = $1.86 | Randomized controlled study with 12 districts as experimental units. HHS and HFS undertaken B&A 2.5 years of implementation | SDC and MC much better than CC. Median double difference on seven indicators for SDC versus CC was 21.3%p for MC versus CC, double difference was 9.3%p | Expanded to twice as many districts |
| 2. Bangladesh rural community nutrition services | SDC with NGOs compared to control areas with no organized nutrition services (i.e., normal government health services with no nutritional component) | 15 million Cost per head per year = $0.96 | Controlled, B&A study with six experimental and two control subdistricts. HHSs conducted by third party | Malnutrition rates declined 18%p in SDC subdistricts compared with 13%p in controls (double difference = 5%p). Double difference for vitamin A was 27%p | Expanded to more than 30 million |
| 3. Bangladesh Urban PHC | SDC with NGOs compared to government provision of services (i.e., CCC) | 4 million Cost per head per year = $0.65 in both SDC and CCC | Controlled B&A study with 15 contracts compared with a large area implemented by CCC. HHS and HFS by third party | Median double difference on 10 HHS indicators was 3.4%p after 2 years. Much larger differences in quality of care indicators from HFS | Contracts not yet completed. Planning for expansion of contracts far advanced and funding secured |
| 4. Bolivia Urban PHC | Limited MC in phase II. MC with expanded authority in phase III. Control area had continued public sector management | 250,000 Cost data not available | Controlled, B&A design, but data from routine reporting system, only few indicators examined | Double difference for deliveries between MC and control was 21%p, 1%p for bed occupancy | Unknown |

*(continued)*

**Table 16.1** (continued)

| Location and type of services (ref) | Type of contract and intervention | Scale and cost | Evaluation methodology | Main results | Subsequent history |
|---|---|---|---|---|---|
| 5. Guatemala Rural PHC in mountainous areas | MC in selected municipalities and SDC in more remote areas, compared to government provision (control) | 3.4 million Cost per head per year = $6.25 | Controlled design based on HHS undertaken by third party 3 years after contracting began | Median difference between MC and control on five indicators was 11%p (range 5–16%p) | Started as small pilot but expanded rapidly. Now covers 27% of the country |
| 6. Haiti bonuses for NGOs delivering PHC in rural areas | NGOs with SDCs offered performance bonuses based on agreed targets | 534,000 Cost data not available | B&A (7 months later) design based on HHSs done by third party | Average of follow-up minus baseline ranged from –3%p (prenatal care) to +32%p (vaccination coverage) | Expanded to cover 3 million people, 33% of the Haitian population |
| 7. India urban TB control services in Hyderabad | NGO under SDC delivered TB control services in defined population and worked with private providers. Compared to publicly managed area of similar size | 500,000 population Cost per patient: SDC = $88, CC = $98 | Controlled design with after-only data from recording system verified by national TB program officials. Cost data obtained by third party | NGO found 2.1% more TB cases and had 1.4%p better treatment success rate. Cost per successful treatment $118 for NGO versus $138 | Being scaled up in various parts of India with continuing evaluation |
| 8. Madagascar and Senegal community nutrition services | Madagascar: SDCs with 50 NGOs Senegal: SDCs with NGOs who worked through small groups of unemployed youth | 460,000 in Madagascar 490,000 in Senegal Cost per beneficiary = $48 and $15, respectively | B&A (17 months) HHS of nutrition status in Senegal. Third-party survey of participation in project and control areas | Severe and moderate malnutrition declined 6%p and 4%p, respectively. Participation was 72% in project and 35% in control areas | Continued with NGOs in both countries, albeit in a different format |

(continued)

**Table 16.1** *(continued)*

| Location and type of services (ref) | Type of contract and intervention | Scale and cost | Evaluation methodology | Main results | Subsequent history |
|---|---|---|---|---|---|
| 9. Pakistan Rural PHC (data obtained by authors) | MC for the 104 basic health units in one district | 3.3 million Cost per head per year = $0.44 | Interrupted time series design based on routine recording and reporting system | Nearly a fourfold increase in the number of outpatient visits | Only started in May 2003 |
| 10. India improving quality of care by private practitioners | SDC for NGO working with private providers to improve MCH services | 54,000 Cost per head per year = $15 | B&A (6 months later) design based on HHS by community health workers | Rapid improvement in provider skills ranging from 25%p to 57%p compared with baseline | Unknown |

*Source:* Loevinsohn and Harding 2005.

MC = management contract, SDC = service delivery contract, CC = control-comparison, double difference = difference between follow-up and baseline results in the experimental group minus the difference between follow-up and baseline results in the control group, B&A = before and after, HHS = household survey, HFS = health facility survey, TB = tuberculosis, NGO = nongovernmental organizations, PHC = primary health care, CCC = Chittagong City Corporation, %p = percentage points, MCH = maternal and child health. All costs are in $U.S. dollars.

***Table 16.2*** *Application of the Concept of Decision Space*

| | Degree of decision space | | |
|---|---|---|---|
| Function | Narrow | Moderate | Wide |
| **Financing** | | | |
| • Sources of revenue | Zambia | Ghana, Uganda | Philippines |
| • Expenditures | | All four | |
| • Income from fees | | Ghana, Uganda, Zambia | |
| **Service organization** | | | |
| • Hospital autonomy | Ghana, Zambia | Uganda | Philippines |
| • Insurance plans | Ghana, Uganda | | Philippines, Zambia |
| • Payment mechanisms | Ghana, Uganda | Philippines | Zambia |
| • Contracts with private providers | | Zambia | Uganda |
| **Human resources** | | | |
| • Salaries | All four | | |
| • Contracts | Ghana | Philippines | Uganda, Zambia |
| • Civil service | Ghana | Philippines, Uganda, Zambia | |
| **Access rules** | Ghana | Philippines, Uganda, Zambia | |
| **Governance** | | | |
| • Local government | Ghana, Zambia | | Philippines, Uganda |
| • Facility boards | All four | | |
| • Health offices | Ghana, Philippines | Uganda, Zambia | |
| • Community participation | Ghana, Uganda | Philippines, Zambia | |

*Source:* Bossert and Beauvais 2002, as reported in Leighton and others 2002.

greater pressure in hiring (because of patronage) and in keeping inefficient facilities open.
- Local demand for quality and access can be more powerfully expressed at local levels, but local managers may go into debt and pass debt on to higher levels.
- Local managers are more likely to be held accountable than distant bureaucrats, but local managers' accountability will depend on who

exercises political power at the local level. In the absence of allocative decision rules set according to national pro-poor directives, local elites may be more effective in pushing for investments in hospitals that benefit the rich than in funding primary care for the poor.

## Typical Decentralization Problems and Some Solutions

Key stakeholders can remedy many of the problems that have emerged during the decentralization process in various countries. But they must recognize and be willing to act on these problems.

One typical problem is that responsibilities are transferred to local units but that the center retains authority over key personnel and budget decisions:

- District health managers are made responsible for health center oversight, but they have limited authority to hire, reward, or sanction center staff.
- Local units are made responsible for health care spending, but they have no revenue-raising authority.
- The center assigns new responsibilities, but provides no additional resources and management authority.

A second problem is that service mix shifts away from priority services. In Honduras, efforts to decentralize Ministry of Health programs led to a decrease in HIV/AIDS surveillance and a significant increase in underreporting of the disease. In Colombia, overall vaccination rates dropped after decentralization, leading to a higher incidence of vaccine-preventable illnesses. Poor capacity for management of an expanded program of immunization and resource competition at local levels were key factors.

These and other problems can be addressed through careful planning and capacity building during the decentralization process. The central government can continue to earmark funds for priority areas, provide guidelines for local priority setting and resource allocation, and maintain central control over critical functions such as procurement and training. As the central government lets go of actual service provision, it can give more attention to oversight, regulation, and stewardship. Some programs—for example, immunizations and malaria control—may require continued central government support for long-term sustainability.

Tracking the impact of all reforms requires identification of winners and losers. During the 1980s, decentralization in Mexico led to some inequitable resource distribution among states. Least developed states had difficulty raising funds to support an insurance program for the poor. Similarly, in

Colombia, localities with greater political influence got a greater share of public resources. Central authorities may need to adjust allocation formulae to ensure that adequate resources can reach poor regions.

Key stakeholders, including the consumers of health services, need information about changes and mechanisms for expressing their concerns to ensure that reforms have the intended positive effects and do not undermine reproductive health and rights. Central governments that relinquish control over the day-to-day business of delivering services can still play a key role in facilitating accountability to stakeholders and in involving them in results assessment and correction of adverse consequences.

# 17

## *Getting It and Spending It Well: Finance Reforms and Reproductive Health*

How much does a given country spend on health? How much should it spend on health? The first question is fairly easy to answer. The World Health Organization maintains databases on health expenditures for most member countries. As table 17.1 shows, the gap in the health spending of low-income countries and that of high-income countries is vast. In 2000 low-income countries (those with less than $1,000 per capita income) spent 3.4 percent of GDP on health on average, while high-income countries (those with over $7,000 per capita income) spent 9.4 percent of GDP on average.

The difference between 3.4 percent and 9.4 percent of GDP hides the real differences in spending when we take into account the magnitudes of GDP for rich and poor countries. On average, low-income countries spend about $8 per capita annually on health, whereas high-income countries spend more than $1,600 per capita annually—*200 times* more than low-income countries. Given this incredible difference in spending, answering the second question of how much should be spent is difficult. Health sector advocates in low- and high-income countries alike feel that not enough is spent on health.

This chapter examines different functions of health sector financing and briefly describes the traditional reform elements of each function as well as recent trends in reform. The aim is to empower reproductive health advocates to engage in finance reform activities to improve reproductive health outcomes.

**Table 17.1** Health Spending by Income Groups and Regions

| Group or region | Total health expenditure (millions) | | Per capita health expenditure | | Share of GDP (%) |
|---|---|---|---|---|---|
| | FX rates | l$ | FX rates | l$ | |
| GDP per capita | | | | | |
| < 1,000 | 3,350 | 9,385 | 8 | 24 | 3.4 |
| 1,000–2,200 | 40,893 | 108,744 | 24 | 65 | 4.5 |
| 2,200–7,000 | 143,510 | 482,515 | 60 | 203 | 5.0 |
| > 7,000 | 2,693,591 | 2,953,025 | 1,686 | 1,849 | 9.4 |
| Region | | | | | |
| Africa | 20,434 | 55,968 | 32 | 88 | 5.5 |
| Americas | 104,073 | 221,613 | 251 | 535 | 7.8 |
| Middle East | 55,765 | 96,525 | 116 | 200 | 4.6 |
| Europe and Central Asia | 37,495 | 115,687 | 106 | 327 | 5.4 |
| OECD | 2,552,728 | 2,650,294 | 2,261 | 2,347 | 9.9 |
| South Asia | 42,727 | 116,879 | 28 | 76 | 4.0 |
| East Asia and Pacific | 68,056 | 296,629 | 46 | 200 | 5.1 |
| Total | 2,881,279 | 3,553,594 | 477 | 589 | 8.1 |

*Source:* Murray and Evans 2003.
*Note:* The columns headed "FX rates" present figures that are converted from local currency into U.S. dollars at official exchange rates. The columns headed "l$" present figures converted from local currency at purchasing power parity rates.

## The Three Functions of Health Finance and Motivations for Their Reform

Health finance has three basic functions: (1) mobilization of revenues for health spending from different sources such as direct and indirect general taxation, earmarked taxation for health, and out-of-pocket spending; (2) pooling of resources; and (3) provider payment.

The most obvious objective of health finance reforms is to improve the health status of the population by increasing the number of people receiving services that address major causes of morbidity and mortality. These services are likely to improve health status only if they are of high quality. Another motivation for finance reforms is to improve equity by ensuring that reforms increase the poorest households' use of health services. Yet another motivation is to address financing inefficiencies so that more people receive services. And still another motivation is to increase resources to the health sector in a sustainable way and to provide a safety net to households by protecting them against catastrophic costs due to illness or injury.

### Resource Mobilization

Traditional ways to collect resources for the health sector include general review taxation, social insurance, and donor project financing. Over the last 10 or so years, newer ways of mobilizing health resources have become popular or have received research and policy attention. Among these relatively new approaches are user fees at public sector facilities, fees for social marketing commodities (such as bed nets and contraceptives), private health insurance, community-based health microinsurance, and new donor financing modalities that support programs rather than projects. Each of the traditional and more recent approaches to revenue generation has attractive features but poses operational challenges.

General government taxation is the most often used source of public sector financing for the health sector. Globally, general taxation accounts for 31 percent of all health spending (figure 17.1). The global numbers largely reflect the way rich countries spend on health.

General review taxes are levied in different ways, and each approach has advantages and disadvantages in terms of equity and efficiency. Economic impacts of different forms of general taxation aside, an important policy variable is the extent of government commitment to the health sector, which is typically measured by the share of total government spending on the health sector.

General tax revenues are generated from a variety of sources. Most countries collect direct and indirect taxes. Direct taxes are personal income taxes, corporate profit taxes, property taxes, and wealth taxes. Indirect taxes are sales taxes, value added taxes, excise taxes (tobacco and alcohol), import duties, and export taxes.

Another traditional form of financing for the health sector is donor financing, typically through project funds for building hospitals, buying drugs or contraceptives, and so on. Recipient countries can make effective use of such limited and limiting financing mechanisms only if they have an overall financing strategy that rationalizes project financing and harmonizes it with national budget financing of the health sector. In the short term, project financing can be useful to bring in capital investments, but it can expose countries to the risk of insufficient financing for the recurrent costs of ensuring returns to the investments.

**Figure 17.1** Composition of World Spending on Health, 2000

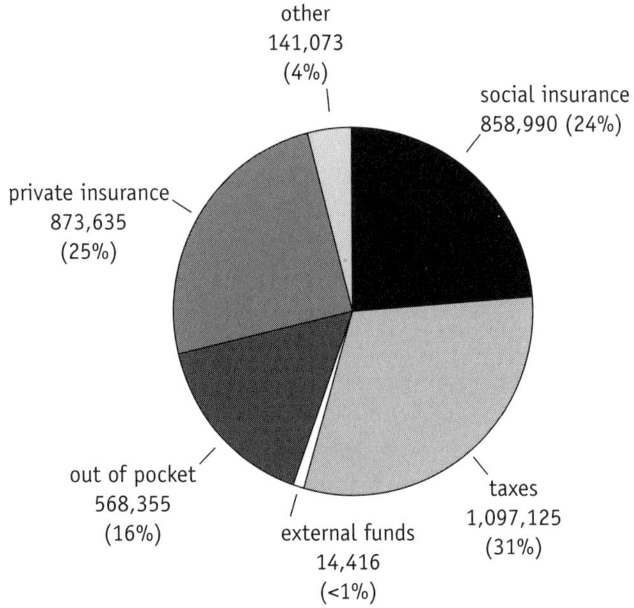

other
141,073
(4%)

social insurance
858,990 (24%)

private insurance
873,635
(25%)

out of pocket
568,355
(16%)

external funds
14,416
(<1%)

taxes
1,097,125
(31%)

*Source:* Murray and Evans 2003.

Social insurance is another traditional source of financing for the health sector, especially in high- and middle-income countries with large formal sectors. Social financing typically involves a law that compels employers to deduct a percentage of each employee's monthly wage for health to be paid to a social insurance fund and that compels employees to pay a percentage of their monthly wage (deducted by the employer) to the fund. Social insurance funds can be managed publicly or privately and can be monopolies or competitively run. The employer/employee deductions are earmarked for health and cannot be used for any other purpose. Such a financing mechanism can only work when employment is largely in the formal sector. A general economic concern about mandatory payroll taxes such as social health insurance is that the compulsory payroll contribution by employers may increase the cost of employing workers. The higher the payroll contribution for health becomes, the more employers will be induced not to hire additional workers. This disincentive may increase unemployment.

A relatively new form of health financing is community-based microinsurance. Community-based fund members voluntarily prepay a set amount each year for a specified package of services. In some cases, governments subsidize the poor if they cannot pay the insurance premium. Typically, the community organizes and operates a primary care clinic at the village level to gain efficiency and quality as well as contracts for secondary services with regional clinics or hospitals. The community manages the fund and is accountable to paying members. The government's role is usually to initiate, train, support, monitor, and regulate the microinsurance schemes.

One of the more controversial approaches to health resource mobilization is user fees (or cost recovery) at public sector clinics. Many countries introduced user fees to raise additional revenue for health and to get consumers to use services more effectively (people value what they pay for and in many cases pay under the table). These fees pose the risk of inequality in access and use of health services. The ideal user fee system ensures that the better off in society are not subsidized for their use of health services, while the poorer segments are not kept away from these services because they cannot afford to pay the fees. Designing and implementing such a system has proven difficult.

## *Pooling Resources*

Pooling describes methods of combining, sharing, and organizing health funds so that the healthy help the sick pay for health care (create a risk pool), and the rich help the poor pay for health care (provide a subsidy to poor).

Traditional forms of resource pooling in the health sector include the budgets of health ministries or other ministries that finance health care (such as armed forces that provide health care to soldiers, veterans, and their families, or education ministries that manage medical schools housed in large hospitals), social security systems (especially in Latin America), and private insurance plans (mostly in high- and middle-income countries). Newer trends in pooling include community-based insurance plans, decentralized district health funds with block grants and basket funds, and combinations of insurance and subsidy pools.

All forms of pooling, including health ministry budgets, incorporate basic elements of insurance and therefore expose the health sector to insurance market failures. One basic insurance question is which services should be covered by insurance. One choice is to insure against uncertain events, such as accidents or catastrophic illnesses, that would expose a patient to considerable expenditures. In this case, a large pool of potential patients may pay a premium, which would cover the costs if they were among the small percentage needing the coverage. In this way, the high costs of treatment would be spread across the whole pool and would financially protect those unlucky few who need the services, as well as buy peace of mind for the insured. Another choice is to insure a basic curative and preventive package of services to ensure that highly cost-effective primary care services reach a large population and minimize the need for more expensive services at a later date.

Another important choice related to pooling is whether to make the decision to join an insurance scheme compulsory (social health insurance) or optional (voluntary private health insurance). Both options have advantages and disadvantages and depend on the nature of the economy and on the capacity of the state to manage or regulate the insurance market. As noted above, social insurance is mainly limited to countries with large formal sectors and can make labor more expensive.

Private voluntary insurance, on the other hand, exposes the health sector to insurance market failures that arise from the asymmetry of information among patients, health providers, and insurance providers. One such potential market failure is moral hazard, or insured consumers' overuse of or demand for health services because they are free.

Another form of market failure is adverse selection, or the likelihood that high-risk patients, more so than low-risk patients, will seek insurance. In other words, people with more current or potential health problems have greater propensity to demand health insurance. Because health insurance companies are unable to distinguish low- from high-risk individuals, they raise their premium, making insurance harder to purchase and compounding the adverse selection problem. As a result of this insurance market failure, the supply of health insurance is insufficient, and without government intervention, some people will be left without insurance protection.

Yet another form of health insurance market failure is risk selection, or attempts of insurers to recruit low-risk patients—also referred to as cherry picking or cream skimming. If insurers manage to, or are allowed to, select the best risks (the young and healthy and men), the elderly, the sick, and women of reproductive age may be left without health insurance coverage.

### Provider Payment

The third function of health financing is provider payment, or the basis on which money is exchanged between parties. How much is paid (or the unit of payment), when payments are made (before or after the service is completed), and the conditions of payment (or the performance criteria) can produce incentives for both payers and providers. Reproductive health advocates who understand these incentives can engage in financing reforms that can improve reproductive health outcomes.

The most typical payment mechanism for facilities is a line item budget allocation to public sector providers. Line items include salaries, capital investments, equipment, medicines, and maintenance. Line item amounts are set on the basis of norms such as number of beds, number of staff, bed occupancy rates, or historic trends. Budget allocations are usually established at the beginning of a fiscal or calendar year to cover services to be provided in that year.

Another traditional form of payment to facilities is grants to nongovernmental organizations (NGOs). These grants are usually provided to increase access to services in geographic regions with few public sector facilities. Such grants take several forms and can be linked to beds or to staff availability, or to the need for drugs or supplies. These grants are made before services are provided and are sometimes linked to expected provision of services to underserved and vulnerable communities. In most cases the payer is the government, but in some countries donors provide direct support to NGOs without going through the health ministry or treasury budget.

Other traditional provider payment tools are retrospective per diem or per admission for inpatient care. In a per diem system, hospitals are paid for each day a patient spends in the hospital. In a per admission system, hospitals are paid for each admission, regardless of how many days the patient stays in the hospital. The systems create different incentives for providers in terms of length of stay and different cost conditions for payers.

Newer trends in provider payment to facilities include attempts to link performance to payment or budgeting, to adjust payment for case severity, or to provide greater autonomy to decentralized structures. In performance-based budgeting, allocations are based on improvements in how facilities deliver services or on the health outcomes that facilities produce. A companion reform is capitation, or less item-specific allocations to block grants that allow facility mangers to make decisions on input mix. Another performance-linked approach to provider payment is contracts with nongovernmental providers. Contracting is becoming more common in the health sector, and the impact of linking outputs to payments is positive (Loevinsohn and Harding 2005).

Many middle-income countries and countries in the Organisation for Economic Co-operation and Development are reimbursing facilities on the basis of severity of the patient's condition. First developed in the United States, diagnostic-related groups (DRGs) define health conditions and possible complications and pay facilities on the basis of the category to which patients are medically assigned.

Traditional approaches to paying individual providers are similar to those for paying facilities. They include salaries or fee for service. Newer approaches include linking payment to performance, severity (DRGs), or capitation.

Analysis of each approach to payment would usually include an assessment of who is bearing the bulk of the financial risks (the patient, the insurer, or the provider); the incentives each method creates for patients, providers, and insurers; how the levels of payments are set (historic, average cost, negotiation, or production estimates); and the expected consequences (in terms of costs, efficiency, quality of care, equity, sustainability, patient satisfaction, and health outcomes). A few of the incentives created by different payment methods are explored below.

An implicit assumption in analyzing incentives created by payment approaches is that providers, insurers, and patients are rational economic actors. Consider responses to a payment method employed by the former Soviet Union and many developing countries: budget transfers based on historic measures of bed occupancy rates. An intelligent hospital administrator would quickly recognize that the budget of the hospital is directly related to keeping beds occupied; as a result patients end up staying in hospitals for long periods. Countries using bed occupancy rates typically have the longest average length of stay per patient in the world.

Now consider the incentives for hospitals and insurers if the dominant payment method is per diem for inpatients. Hospitals would extend the length of stay in the realization that additional days in the hospital for mostly cured patients are not very costly to the hospital but that each additional day adds to the bill the insurance company pays. Insurance companies, on the other hand, would put pressure on hospitals to reduce the number of days a patient spends in the hospital.

Provider payment methods can produce incentives to change number of services provided, number of patients served, length of stay in hospitals, clinical quality of care, service quality of care, patient referral patterns, and patient population served.

## Health Financing Reforms and Reproductive Health

How can the reproductive health community engage in health financing reform to maximize the benefits of the reform effort and to mitigate any negative impacts on the reproductive health agenda in a given country?

The first step is to better understand the motivation for finance reforms as well as the options under consideration. As noted above, the motivation for reform is improving health outcomes, typically through increased availability of the appropriate services delivered efficiently, equitably, and sustainably. Therefore, reproductive health advocates should ensure that health sector finance reform is focused on reproductive health outcomes (for example, maternal mortality and fertility) and that reproductive health services will be made available to the populations that need them most. Reproductive health, along with child health and nutrition, should be the driver of finance reform and a measure of how success and failure are measured.

After ensuring that the objective of finance reform is addressing reproductive health needs, reproductive health advocates should analyze the possible impact of the different options under consideration. A basic framework for this work follows.

### *Equity and Access*

Mobilization    What are the effects of various mobilization strategies on use of critical health services (including reproductive health services) by different socioeconomic and demographic groups? Stated differently, who bears the burden of paying for health services, and do incentives encourage or discourage service use? How do different mobilization strategies affect service affordability for households at different socioeconomic levels?

Pooling    Whom (for example, the poor and women of reproductive age) do pooled resources cover? Can subsidies and waivers for target groups be included? Does the pooling mechanism limit or expand consumer choice?

Provider Payment    Are the incentives to providers designed to increase or decrease the provision of reproductive health services, especially for the poor and vulnerable (for example, higher capitation for underserved populations/areas)? Are the incentives to patients designed to increase or decrease the demand for reproductive health services, especially by the poor and vulnerable?

### Quality

Mobilization    Do reforms raise enough revenue to maintain or improve quality? Are the revenues mobilized at the facility or community level recycled to improve quality?

Pooling    Do service packages funded through the pooling mechanism include reproductive health services? Do financial arrangements permit coverage and provision of priority reproductive health services?

Provider Payment    Are providers rewarded for provision of high-quality services? Do the payment mechanisms empower payers (patients or insurers) to insist on high-quality services?

### Efficiency

Mobilization    Are reforms likely to encourage people to underuse or overuse health services?

Pooling    What is the relative complexity and cost of administrative requirements? Data collection? Consumer education?

Provider Payment    Are providers pressured to cut costs? Are they encouraged to waste resources?

### Sustainability

Mobilization    Will reforms increase or decrease health-spending gaps? Are they affordable to all main fund sources?

Pooling    Does the community participate in and trust the pooling institution? What is the risk pool's viable size? What is the insurability of covered services?

Provider Payment    Do payment mechanisms create incentives for sustainable payment levels?

  Armed with answers to these questions, champions of reproductive health can influence how resources are mobilized, pooled, and spent.

# Notes

1. See UNFPA 2005.

2. A possible exception would be family planning services, especially those delivered through outreach mechanisms.

3. See chapter 4 for an analysis of global trends in aid modalities and chapters 15–17 for an analysis of health sector reform and strengthening.

4. The PROFILES computer program is based on scientific knowledge about the returns to nutrition interventions. Many countries have used the program in making the economic and health argument for public investments.

5. Some progress is being made, for example, with gender-specific versions of the Human Development Index (HDI).

6. It should be noted that, despite the greater attention to reproductive ill health in the second round of the burden of disease exercise in 1999, codes 9 and 10 of the International Classification of Diseases omit both female genital mutilation and contraceptive morbidity.

7. We employ the terms "north" and "south" to characterize this broad division rather than terms like "more developed" or "less developed." Neither breakdown is adequate, but the former is a convenient way of separating countries whose demographic transitions occurred earlier from countries where transitions came later.

8. In 1997, according to UNFPA and UNAIDS, 41 percent of adults living with HIV/AIDS worldwide were women. By 2001 this figure had risen to 50 percent. By late 2005, women in Sub-Saharan Africa accounted for nearly 60 percent of new infections.

9. Globally, approximately 70 percent of HIV infections occur as a result of hetero-sexual intercourse; in Sub-Saharan Africa, this proportion reaches 90 percent.

10. Data were compiled by the Division for the Advancement of Women, United Nations.

11. Even in countries where European Union or other laws apply, the pay gap remains. Among the reasons is reluctance on the part of many women to take their employers to court because they fear further discrimination.

12. Much of this section is reproduced from the overview of the 2005 UNICEF report, "Female Genital Mutilation/Cutting—A Statistical Exploration," available at http://www.unicef.org/publications/index_29994.html.

13. Girls' attendance at school is at times also constrained by the lack of latrines or running water at school, which is especially important after girls start menstruating.

14. . . . but please take these characterizations with a grain of salt. No disrespect of any of the players in the prioritization process is intended.

15. The most popular epidemiological tools for measuring burden of disease are years of life lost (YLL), disability adjusted life years (DALY) and quality adjusted life years (QALY).

16. See Drummond (1987).

17. The international health community recently coined a term—international public goods—that mixes externalities and public goods. In essence, international public goods are the services that address large social and cross-border externalities, such as communicable diseases, even though these services are private in nature.

18. A review of more than 100 published articles and books on prioritization and resource allocation in the health sector found little agreement on the best way to move forward. Some telling titles are "Reluctant Rationers" and "No Easy Choices."

19. This section relies heavily on Bitran (1998), which relied heavily on Cumming (1994).

20. The poor suffer disproportionately from all types of diseases, but the burden of communicable disease, what public health specialists refer to as the unfinished agenda, falls mainly on the poorest people.

21. As some researchers have noted (McCarthy 1997; Thaddeus and Maine 1994), the empirical evidence on links between maternal education and use of health services is not at all clear-cut. Some educated women may choose to rely on self-care and self-medication and to postpone visits to a facility until after such methods fail. If education is associated with a desire for fewer births and later marriage, there may be more unintended pregnancies and higher abortion rates, which would pose greater risk when access to safe abortion is limited.

22. For examples of good social conditions in Scandinavia and Europe generally, see T. R. Reid, *The United States of Europe*, 2004.

23. Kerala's MMR of 87 is less than a sixth of India's national average and less than an eighth of the rate in Orissa in the country's north.

24. The model is based on cross-national regression analyses of MMRs; the percentage of GDP is expanded on health and other variables, including government effectiveness, female education, and water supply. The methodology and regression analyses are explained in annex 2 of Wagstaff and Claeson (2004).

25. Situational factors may be considered short term, whereas structural factors are long term. However, rapid political changes and global communications have blurred this distinction.

26. The World Bank Institute's program on Reproductive Health and Health Sector Reform, developed in 1998, is offered in locations around the world. Participants in these courses include government officials from the health and planning ministries, civil society representatives, academicians, and staff from bilateral and multilateral agencies. See www.worldbank.org/wbi/healthandpopulation.

27. An excellent treatment of health sector reform exists in Roberts and others (2004).

28. For a detailed discussion of decentralization and reproductive health, see Aitken (1998).

29. Zambia's experience is documented in Nanda (2000).

30. See Standing (1997) for an extensive review of the effects of user fees and other reforms.

31. See Diop, Yazbeck, and Bitrán (1995).

32. See Ddymtraczenko (1998).

33. See Corrêa, Pilla, and Arilha (1998).

34. The World Health Organization has proposed a set of reproductive health indicators (WHO 1997). Although not specifically focused on reproductive health, a good overview of issues in evaluating health reforms can be found in McPake and Kutzin (1997).

# Bibliography

Ahlburg, D. A. 2002. "Does Population Matter? A Review Essay." *Population and Development Review* 28(2): 329–50.

Ahluwalia, I. B., T. Schmidt, and others. 2003. "An Evaluation of a Community-Based Approach to Safe Motherhood in Northwestern Tanzania." *International Journal of Gynecology and Obstetrics* 82: 231–40.

Aitken, Iain. 1998. "Implications of Decentralization as a Reform Strategy for the Implementation of Reproductive Health Programs." In *Report of the Meeting on the Implications of Health Sector Reform on Reproductive Health and Rights.* Washington, DC: Center for Health and Gender Equity/The Population Council.

Askew, I., and M. Berer. 2003. "The Contribution of Sexual and Reproductive Health Services to the Fight against HIV/AIDS: A Review." *Reproductive Health Matters* 11: 51–73.

Beegle, K., E. Frankenberg, and D. Thomas. 2001. "Bargaining Power within Couples and Use of Prenatal and Delivery Care in Indonesia." *Studies in Family Planning* 32(2): 130–146.

Berman, Peter A. 1995. "Health Sector Reform: Making Health Development Sustainable." In *Health Sector Reform in Developing Countries*, ed. Peter A. Behman. Cambridge: Harvard University Press.

Birdsall, N., A. C. Kelley, and others, eds. 2001. *Population Matters: Demographic Change, Economic Growth, and Poverty in the Developing World.* Oxford: Oxford University Press.

Bitrán y Asociados. 1998. "Designing a Benefits Package." Unpublished paper prepared for Flagship Course on Health Sector Reform and Sustainable Financing, World Bank Institute, Washington DC.

Blackden, C. M., and C. Bhanu. 1999. "Gender, Growth and Poverty Reduction. Special Program of Assistance for Africa, 1998 Status Report on Poverty." Technical Paper No. 428. World Bank, Washington, DC.

Blanchet, T. 1991. "Maternal Health in Rural Bangladesh." Bangladesh Country Office, UNICEF, Dhaka.

Bloom, D. E., D. Canning, and others. 2004. "Health, Wealth, and Welfare." *Finance and Development* 41(1): 10–15.

Bossert, T., and J. Beauvais. 2002. "Decentralization of Health Systems in Ghana, Zambia, Uganda, and the Philippines: A Comparative Analysis of Decision Space." *Health Policy and Planning* 17 (1): 14–31.

Brinkerhoff, Derick W., and Benjamin L. Crosby. 2002. *Managing Policy Reform: Concepts and Tools for Decision-Makers in Developing and Transition Countries.* Bloomfield: Kumarian Press.

Buckshee, K. 1997. "Impact of Roles of Women on Health in India." *International Journal of Gynecology and Obstetrics* 58: 35–42.

Case, A., and A. Deaton. 2002. "Consumption, Health, Gender and Poverty." Research Program in Development Studies, Princeton University, Princeton, New Jersey.

Castro-Leal, F., and others. 1999. "Public Social Spending in Africa: Do the Poor Benefit?" *The World Bank Research Observer* 14(1): 49–72.

CIET (Community Information, Empowerment and Transparency)-Canada. 2001. Health and population sector programme, 1998–2003. Service Delivery Survey, Second Cycle. Ministry of Health and Family Welfare, Dhaka.

Claeson, M., and C. Griffin, T. Johnston, M. McLachlan, A. Soucat, A. Wagstaff, and A. Yazbeck. 2002. "Health, Nutrition and Population." In J. Klugman, ed., *A Sourcebook for Poverty Reduction Strategies,* vol. 2. Washington, DC: The World Bank.

Corrêa, Sonia, Sérgio Pilla, and Margareth Arilha. 1998. *Reproductive Health in Policy and Practice: Brazil.* Washington, DC: Population Reference Bureau.

Cummings, J. 1994. "Core Services and Priority Setting: The New Zealand Experience." *Health Policy* 29: 41–60.

Ddymtraczenko, Tania. 1998. "Evaluation of the National Mother-Child Health Insurance Program in Bolivia." Available at http://www.phrproject.com/publicat/inbriefs/ib20fin.htm.

Diop, François, Abdo Yazbeck, and Ricardo Bitrán. 1995. "The Impact of Alternative Cost Recovery Schemes on Access and Equity in Niger." *Health Policy and Planning* 10: 223–40.

Douki, D., and others. 2003. *Violence against Women in Arabic and Islamic Countries.* Faculty of Medicine of Tunis, Tunis, Tunisia.

Elsen, Diane, Barbara Evers, and Jasmine Gideon. 1998. "Whys and Hows of Gender Aware Country Economic Reports." *ICDA Journal, Focus on Trade and Development* 6 (1): 26.

El-Zanaty, F., E. Hussein, G. A. Shawky, A. A. Way, and S. Kishor. 1996. *Egypt Demographic and Health Survey 1995.* Calverton, Md.: Macro International, Inc.

Ensor, T., and S. Cooper. 2004. "Overcoming Barriers to Health Service Access: Influencing the Demand Side." *Health Policy and Planning* 19(2): 69–79.

Epstein, B. 2004. "The Demographic Import of HIV/AIDS" in M. Haacker, ed., *The Macronomics of HIV/AIDS.* Washington, DC: International Monetary Fund.

Essien, E., D. Ifenne, and others. 1997. "Community Loan Funds and Transport Services for Obstetric Emergencies in Northern Nigeria." *International Journal of Gynecology and Obstetrics* 69 Supplement (2): S237–44.

Family Care International and the Safe Motherhood Inter-Agency Group. 1998. "Improving Access to Maternal Health Services." Fact sheet.

Fawcus, S., M. Mbviso, and others. 1996. "A Community-Based Investigation of Avoidable Factors for Maternal Mortality in Zimbabwe." *Studies in Family Planning* 27(6): 319–27.

Filmer, Deon. 2003. "The Incidence of Public Expenditures on Health and Development." Background note for *World Development Report 2004.* World Bank, Washington, DC.

Filmer, Deon, and Lant H. Pritchett. 2001. "Estimating Wealth Effects without Expenditure Data—or Tears: An Application to Educational Enrollments in States of India." *Demography* 38: 115–32.

Germain A. 2003. "Making the Link: Sexual and Reproductive Health and Health Systems." Keynote speech at Making the Link: Sexual-Reproductive Health and Health Systems, Leeds, September 9–11.

Gillespie, D. 2003. "Whatever Happened to Family Planning?" Presentation to the David and Lucile Packard Foundation.

Gilson, L. 1997. "The Lessons of User Fee Experience in Africa: Review Paper." *Health Policy and Planning* 12(4): 273–85.

Girard, F. 2001. "Reproductive Health Under Attack at the United Nations" (letter). *Reproductive Health Matters* 9: 68.

Granstrom, O. and A. Yazbeck. 2006, "An Idiot's Guide to Global Health Initiatives." Unpublished report.

Gwatkin D. 2002. "Overcoming the Inverse Care Law." Leverhulme Lecture, London School of Tropical Medicine, September.

Gwatkin, D., and others. 2000. Socioeconomic Differences in Health, Nutrition, and Population. Washington DC: World Bank, Health, Nutrition, and Population Department.

Gwatkin, D., A. Wagstaff, and A. Yazbeck 2005. *Reaching the Poor with Health, Nutrition, and Population Services.* Washington, DC: International Bank for Reconstruction and Development.

Hall, P. E., and C. Chhoung. 2005. "Reproductive Health Commodity Security Country Case Study: Cambodia." Unpublished report. DFID Health Resource Centre.

Inter-Parliamentary Union. 2001. *Women in Parliament in 2001: The Year in Perspective.* Geneva.

Jahan R. 2003. "Sustaining Advocacy for the ICPD Agenda in Health Reforms under Regime Change: Lessons from Bangladesh." Presentation at Making the Link: Sexual-Reproductive Health and Health Systems, Leeds, September 9–11.

Jalan, J., and M. Ravallion. 2001. "Does Piped Water Reduce Diarrhea for Children in Rural India?" Policy Research Paper 2664. World Bank, Washington, DC.

Jejeebhoy, S. 1995. *Women's Education, Autonomy, and Reproductive Behaviour: Experience from Developing Countries.* Oxford: Clarendon Press.

Jejeebhoy, S., M. A. Koenig, and others. 2003. *Reproductive Tract Infections and Other Gynaecological Disorders: Research into Prevalence, Correlates, and Consequences.* Cambridge: Cambridge University Press.

Kaufmann, D., A. Kraay, and others. 2003. "Government Matters III: Governance Indicators for 1996–2002." World Bank, Washington, DC.

King, R., J. Estey, S. Allen, S. Kegeles, W. Wolf, C. Valentine, and A. Serufilira. 1995. "A Family Planning Intervention to Reduce Vertical Transmission of HIV in Rwanda." *AIDS* 9 Suppl 1: S45-51.

Knowles, J. 2000. "Benefit Incidence Analysis of Safe Motherhood Services in Vietnam." Paper prepared for WBI Core Course. World Bank Institute, Washington DC.

Krasovec K., and R. P. Shaw. 2000. "Reproductive Health and Health Sector Reform: Linking Outcomes to Action." Draft paper for Module 7, Core Course, Adapting to Change: Population, Reproductive Health, and Health Sector Reform, World Bank Institute, Washington DC.

Kunst, A. E., and T. Houweling. 2001. "A Global Picture of Poor-Rich Differences in the Utilization of Delivery Care." *Studies in Health Services and Organisation and Policy* 17: 293–311.

Lakshminarayanan. R. 2003. "Decentralization and Its Implications for Reproductive Health: The Philippines Experience." *Reproductive Health Matters 2003* 11 (21): 96–107.

Lalonde, A. B., P. Okong, and others. 2003. "The FIGO Save the Mothers Initiative: Uganda-Canada Collaboration." *International Journal of Gynecology and Obstetrics* 80 204–12.

Leighton, C., and D. Brinkerhoff. 2002. *Decentralization and Health Sector Reform.* Insights for Implementers series. Bethesda, Md: Partners for Health Reformplus, Abt Associates Inc.

Link, B. G., and J. C. Phelan. 2002. "McKeown and the Idea That Social Conditions Are Fundamental Causes of Disease." *American Journal of Public Health* 92 (5): 730–32.

Loevinsohn, B., and A. Harding. 2005. "Buying Results? Contracting for Health Service Delivery in Developing Countries." *Lancet* 366: 676–81.

Lule, E. 2004. "Strengthening the Linkages between Reproductive Health and HIV/AIDS Programs." Unpublished report, Human Development Network, World Bank, Washington, DC.

Malhotra, A., and others. 2005. "Nepal: The Distributional Impact of Participatory Approaches on Reproductive Health for Disadvantaged Youth." In *Reaching the Poor with Health, Nutrition, and Population Services*, ed. D. Gwatkin, A. Wagstaff, and A. Yazbeck. Washington, DC: World Bank.

Mason, A. 2001. *Population Change and Economic Development in East Asia: Challenges Met, Opportunities Seized*. Stanford, Calif.: Stanford University Press.

McCarthy, J. 1997. "The Conceptual Framework of the PMM Network." *International Journal of Gynecology and Obstetrics* 59 Suppl.: S15–21.

McPake, Barbara, and Joseph Kutzin. 1997. "Methods for Evaluating Effects of Health Reforms." Research and Assessment Paper 13, Division of Analysis, World Health Organization, Geneva.

Merrick, T. 2005. "Maternal-Neonatal Health (MNH) and Poverty: Factors beyond Care That Affect MNH Outcomes" Geneva: World Health Organization.

Mirembe, Florence, Freddie Ssengooba, and Rosalind Lubanga. 1998. *Reproductive Health in Policy and Practice: Uganda*. Washington, DC: Population Reference Bureau.

Murray, Christopher and David Evans, eds. 2003. *Health System Performance Assessment*. Geneva: World Health Organization.

Nahar, S., and A. Costello. 1998. "The Hidden Cost of 'Free' Maternity Care in Dhaka, Bangladesh." *Health Policy and Planning* 13(4): 417–22.

Nanda, Priya. 2000. "Health Sector Reform in Zambia: Trade-offs for the Reproductive Health and Rights Agenda." Working paper, Center for Health and Gender Equity, Washington, DC.

Newbrander, W., D. Collins, and others. 2000. *Ensuring Equal Access to Health Services: User Fee Systems and the Poor.* Boston: Management Sciences for Health.

Newman, J., M. Pradhan, and others. 2002. "An Impact Evaluation of Education, Health, and Water Supply Investments by the Bolivian Social Investment Fund." *World Bank Economic Review* 16(2): 241–74.

Pathmanathan, I., J. Liljestrand, and others. 2003. "Investing in Maternal Health: Learning from Malaysia and Sri Lanka." Human Development Network, World Bank, Washington, DC.

Paul, B. K. 1993. "Maternal Mortality in Africa: 1980–87." *Social Science and Medicine* 37(6): 745–52.

Peters, David H., Abdo S. Yazbeck, Rashmi R. Sharma , G. N. V. Ramana, Lant H. Pritchett, Adam Wagstaff. 2002. *Better Health Systems for India's Poor: Findings, Analysis, and Options.* Washington, DC: World Bank

Population Action International. 2001. *Overview: The need for security in reproductive health services. Meeting the Challenge.* http://www.populationaction.org/resources/publications/commodities/PDFs/PAI_02_Eng.pdf

Population Reference Bureau. 2004. "Transitions in World Population." *Population Bulletin* 59(1): 13.

Ratzan S, G. Filerman, and J. Lesar. 2000. "Attaining Global Health: Challenges and Consequences." *Population Bulletin* 55(1): 1–48.

Rawlings, Laura, Lynne Sherburne-Benz, and Julie Van Domelen. 2004. *Evaluating Social Funds: A Cross-Country Analysis of Community Investments. Regional and Sectoral Studies.* Washington, DC: World Bank.

Reid, T. 2004. *The United States of Europe.* New York: Penguin Group.

Roberts, M. J., and others. 2004. *Getting Health Reform Right: A Guide to Improving Performance and Equity.* Oxford: Oxford University Press.

Rutstein, S. 2000. "Effects of Birth Interval on Mortality and Health: Multivariate Cross-Country Analysis." Presentation to USAID. MACRO International.

Samai, O., and P. Sengeh. 1997. "Facilitating Emergency Obstetric Care through Transportation and Communication, Bo, Sierra Leone." *International Journal of Gynecology and Obstetrics* 59(Suppl. 2): S157–64.

Santiso, R. 1997. "Effects of Chronic Parasitosis on Women's Health." *International Journal of Gynecology and Obstetrics* 58: 129–36.

Schultz, T. P. 2004. "Demographic Determinants of Savings: Estimating and Interpreting the Aggregate Association in Asia." Discussion Paper 901, Economic Growth Center, Yale University, New Haven, Connecticut.

Schwartz, J.B., and Bhushan, I. 2005. "Cambodia: Using Contracting to Reduce Inequity in Primary Health Care Delivery." In *Reaching the Poor with Health, Nutrition, and Population Services*, ed. D. Gwatkin, A. Wagstaff, and A. Yazbeck. Washington, DC: International Bank for Reconstruction and Development.

Soucat, A., and others. 2002. "Marginal Budgeting for Bottlenecks: A New Costing and Resource Allocation Practice to Buy Health Results." Policy and Sector Analysis Support Team, Africa Region Human Development, World Bank, Washington, DC.

Standing, Hilary. 1997. "Gender and Equity in Health Sector Reform Programmes: A Review." *Health Policy and Planning* 12: 1–18.

Stover, J. 2003. "Cost and Benefits of Providing Family Planning Services at PMTCT and VCT Sites." Unpublished.

Sundari, T. 1992. "The Untold Story: How the Health Care Systems in Developing Countries Contribute to Maternal Mortality." *International Journal of Health Services* 22(3): 513–28.

Thaddeus, S., and D. Maine. 1994. "Too Far to Walk: Maternal Mortality in Context." *Social Science and Medicine* 38(8): 1091–110.

UNDP (United Nations Development Program). 1998. Benin—Time Allocation Study. New York: UNDP.

———. 2003. *Human Development Report 2003.* New York: UNDP.

UNFPA (United Nations Population Fund). 2005. *State of World Population 2005: The Promise of Equality: Gender Equity, Reproductive Health and the Millennium Development Goals.* New York: UNFPA.

UNICEF (United Nations Children's Fund). 2005. "Female Genital Mutilation/Cutting—A Statistical Exploration." Available at www.unicef.org/publications/index_29994.html.

United Nations. 1995. *Programme of Action Adopted at International Conference on Population and Development*, Cairo, 5-13 September 1994, para. 7-2. UN, New York

———. 1996. *World Population Prospects: The 1996 Revision.* Annex I: Demographic Indicators. Department for Economic and Social Information and Policy Analysis, Population Division, United Nations, New York.

———. 1998a. *World Population Prospects: The 1998 Revision.* Annex I: Demographic Indicators. Department for Economic and Social Information and Policy Analysis, Population Division, United Nations, New York.

———. 1998b. *World Population Projections to 2150.* Department for Economic and Social Information and Policy Analysis, Population Division, United Nations, New York.

USAID. "Policy Toolkit for Strengthening Health Sector Reform." Partners for Health Reform Project, Washington, DC.

van Poppel, F., and C. van der Heijden. 1997. "The Effects of Water Supply on Infant and Child Mortality: A Review of Historical Evidence." *Health Transition Review* 7(2): 113–48.

Wagstaff, A., and M. Claeson. 2004. *The Millennium Development Goals for Health: Rising to the Challenges.* Washington, DC: The World Bank.

Walt, G., and L. Gilson. 1994. "Reforming the Health Sector in Developing Countries: The Central Role of Policy Analysis." *Health Policy and Planning* 9: 353–70.

Westoff, C. 2003. "Analysis of Selected DHS Data." Unpublished.

WHO (World Health Organization). 1997. *Monitoring Reproductive Health: Selecting a Short List of National and Global Indicators*. Geneva: WHO.

———. 1999. *World Health Report*. Geneva: WHO.

———. 2003. Pregnancy, Childbirth, Postpartum and Newborn Care: A Guide for Essential Practice. Geneva: WHO.

Wilson, E. 2000. "Implications of Decentralization for Reproductive Health Planning in Senegal." *Policy Matters* No. 3. The Policy Project, Washington, DC.

World Bank. 1996. "Kingdom of Morocco: Impact Evaluation Report: Socioeconomic Influence of Rural Roads." Operations Evaluation Department, World Bank, Washington, DC.

———. 2003a. "Poverty Reduction in Guatemala." Poverty and Economic Management Unit, Latin America and the Caribbean Region, World Bank, Washington DC.

———. 2003b. *World Development Report 2004: Making Services Work for Poor People*. Washington, DC: World Bank.

# Index